Breast Cytopathology

Monographs in Clinical Cytology

Vol. 24

Series Editor

Philippe Vielh Dudelange, Luxembourg

Maurizio Pinamonti Trieste
Fabrizio Zanconati Trieste

Breast Cytopathology

Assessing the Value of FNAC in the Diagnosis of Breast Lesions

126 figures, 119 in color, 2018

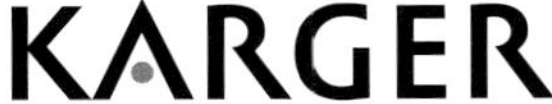
Basel · Freiburg · Paris · London · New York · Chennai · New Delhi · Bangkok · Beijing · Shanghai · Tokyo · Kuala Lumpur · Singapore · Sydney

Monographs in Clinical Cytology
Founded 1965 by Georg L. Wied, Chicago, IL

Dr. Maurizio Pinamonti
Department of Medical Sciences
University of Trieste
IT--34149 Trieste (Italy)

Prof. Fabrizio Zanconati
Department of Medical Sciences
University of Trieste
IT--34149 Trieste (Italy)

Library of Congress Cataloging-in-Publication Data

Names: Pinamonti, Maurizio, author. | Zanconati, Fabrizio, author.
Title: Breast cytopathology : assessing the value of FNAC in the diagnosis of breast lesions / Maurizio Pinamonti, Fabrizio Zanconati.
Other titles: Monographs in clinical cytology ; v. 24.
Description: Basel ; New York : Karger, 2018. | Series: Monographs in clinical cytology ; vol. 24 | Includes index.
Identifiers: LCCN 2017046399| ISBN 9783318061406 (hard cover : alk. paper) | ISBN 9783318061413 (electronic version)
Subjects: | MESH: Breast--pathology | Breast Diseases--diagnosis | Biopsy, Fine-Needle | Breast Neoplasms--diagnosis
Classification: LCC RG493.5.B56 | NLM WP 815 | DDC 618.1/90758--dc23 LC record available at https://lccn.loc.gov/2017046399

Bibliographic Indices. This publication is listed in bibliographic services, including Current Contents®.

www.karger.com
Printed on acid-free and non-aging paper (ISO 9706)
ISSN 0077–0809
ISBN 978–3–318–06140–6
e-ISBN 978–3–318–06141–3

Contents

Preface

Antoine Zajdela would be happy to see the birth of a text atlas of breast cytopathology realized by one of his Italian students who followed with great interest the courses he held annually in Italy in the 1980s and 1990s. Fabrizio Zanconati, besides being a regular attendant, was among the most interested, assimilating from the teacher not only his diagnostic rigor but also the same enthusiasm. Over the years, he has always cultivated this branch of cytopathology becoming the backbone of breast screening in the Province of Trieste. His enthusiasm brought him alongside with the radiologists attending each breast examination that required a deepening through fine-needle aspiration, which he performed firsthand. This allowed him to merge the microscopic evaluation with clinical information, bringing him to a perfect detection and understanding of breast pathology.

His results are the testimony of his great work, and this text atlas, written with Maurizio Pinamonti, educated at the Trieste Cytopathology School, is its fruit. A clear and precise work that will be of great help to those who approach the diagnosis of breast diseases and that will convince even the most skeptical, who prefer other approaches, to the use of cytology diagnostics.

Luigi Di Bonito, Trieste

Pinamonti M, Zanconati F: Breast Cytopathology. Assessing the Value of FNAC in the Diagnosis of Breast Lesions.
Monogr Clin Cytol. Basel, Karger, 2018, vol 24, pp 1–8 (DOI: 10.1159/000479762)

FNAC: Sampling and Preparation Technique, Fixation, and Staining

What Is FNAC?

Fine-needle aspiration cytology (FNAC) is generally considered a rapid, reliable, safe diagnostic procedure to obtain cellular samples of a lesion via insertion of a thin needle (23–27 G) for subsequent microscopic analysis. It is widely used in a variety of fields and, above all, for superficial palpable masses like many breast lesions. However, under instrumental guidance, FNAC can also be performed on nonpalpable masses; the use of ultrasound guidance largely improves its accuracy in breast diagnostics, reducing sampling errors and avoiding complications [Liao et al., 2004].

In developed countries, mammographic screening programs have been used extensively to detect breast cancer as early as possible in the last 20 years. This resulted in the detection of an increasing number of nonpalpable suspicious or doubtful breast lesions for further investigation. The FNAC report is extremely important because it provides necessary information for the management of patients, i.e., whether to proceed with more invasive diagnostic methods or surgical treatment or not, and helps to decide what kind of operation to perform.

Compared to other more invasive diagnostic techniques, such as core needle biopsy (CNB) and surgical excision, FNAC has many advantages, which are briefly listed below [Zajdela et al., 1995]:

- The examination is easy to perform and quick, requiring few minutes from the time the patient is placed on the bed to the completion of the samples
- The puncture is usually not painful, thus no anesthetic is required due to the small size of the needles, which are even thinner than those used to deliver anesthetics
- It is possible to immediately evaluate the adequacy of the sample and even hypothesize a first diagnosis by the rapid on-site evaluation (ROSE; see below), and thus an immediate repetition of the examination in case of scant or unsatisfactory material is possible
- The fine needle does not cause large tissue damage or serious hemorrhage, side effects such as hematoma formation and pneumothorax are minimized, and in the case of an eventual surgical resection of the lesion, tissue quality is preserved
- By moving the needle inside the lesion during the aspiration, it is possible to sample different lesion parts, potentially improving sensitivity

- The examiner's hand has tactile perception of the consistence of the lesion
- It is possible to examine several different lesions and axillary lymph nodes in the same session
- In the case of liquid lesions, the examination becomes potentially therapeutic, i.e., cysts may be emptied
- The cost of the procedure is low compared to other diagnostic techniques

Cytology has indeed some limitations; it does not allow an accurate evaluation of tissue architecture even if cells tend to maintain the way they are connected to each other on cytological smears. Some sclerotic or poorly cellular lesions often give unsatisfactory results, and the number of special stains is limited. However, it is possible to collect material for immunocytochemistry by preparing multiple slides from the same lesion or using liquid-based cytology or cell block techniques [Domanski et al., 2013; Ferguson et al., 2013; Garbar and Curé, 2013]. Moreover, FNAC is able to provide optimal material to perform molecular analyses on cancer cells.

Most of the criticism leveled at FNAC is due to its high rate of unsatisfactory examinations [Willems et al., 2012], but this is not the case in every laboratory. FNAC is a specialized technique that needs specific skills to be properly performed and interpreted. The reliability and efficiency of the method depend on the quality of the samples and the experience of the medical staff that performs the aspiration [Zagorianakou et al., 2005]. To get the best results, every single step from sampling to spreading and fixation must be correctly performed. In laboratories with little experience in the field of cytology, CNB should be preferred as first-line diagnostic technique.

In institutions with qualified personnel experienced in FNAC, CNB and FNAC can play a complementary role to correctly identify the vast majority of breast lesions without the need of surgical diagnostic biopsies or frozen sections. The decision to use either FNAC or CNB to obtain a definitive diagnosis before operation/treatment is an essential step in the approach to breast carcinoma management at present [Kocjan et al., 2008].

Performing FNAC

FNAC is an ambulatory procedure that requires equipment that is readily available in most health institutions. Many pathology departments comprise a clinic where pathologists themselves perform the aspirates, although a large number of cytology slides come from other clinics where general practitioners, radiologists, or other health care workers perform the examinations. In general, samples have a higher quality and a lower rate of inadequacy when the aspirates are performed by trained cytopathologists in specialized breast clinics [Vural et al., 1995]. Theoretically, the examination may be conducted by a single practitioner, but the ideal situation is the one in which a radiologist, a nurse, and a cytopathologist work together in the same room.

The minimum requirement (Fig. 1) to obtain an aspirate is:

- 23- to 27-G sterile disposable needles
- 10- to 20-mL sterile syringes
- Gloves
- Cotton and antiseptic solution – for quick antisepsis of the skin above the lesion
- Glass slides for smear preparation – they should be marked with the patient's name and/or an identification number
- Liquid fixatives (preferably 95% alcohol) – for Papanicolaou staining

Other equipment that could be useful in specific situations is:

- Syringe holder for the aspiration procedure
- Flexible connector
- Reagents for rapid staining
- Coverslips for the immediate preparation of stained slides
- Microscope – to allow ROSE
- Sterile tubes for bacteriology
- Vials for liquid-based cytology or cell block preparations

The FNAC procedure has some minor differences depending on the technique the examiner is most confident with and on the availability of the personnel. Whatever the technique chosen, the aim of FNAC is to sample large parts of the lesion by means of multidirectional movements of the needle, gathering cell-rich material, and causing the least tissue damage possible. Note that the cytological material should fill just the lumen or the cone of the needle, with the exception of cystic lesions, from which a large amount of liquid material can be drained. The presence of blood impairs the interpretation of the sample, so if blood becomes visible in the cone of the needle, the procedure must be immediately interrupted, and the needle retracted. Waste of potentially diagnostic material must be avoided, however, and thus the collected material should be used anyway, even if it is bloody, but another sampling is highly recommended in these cases.

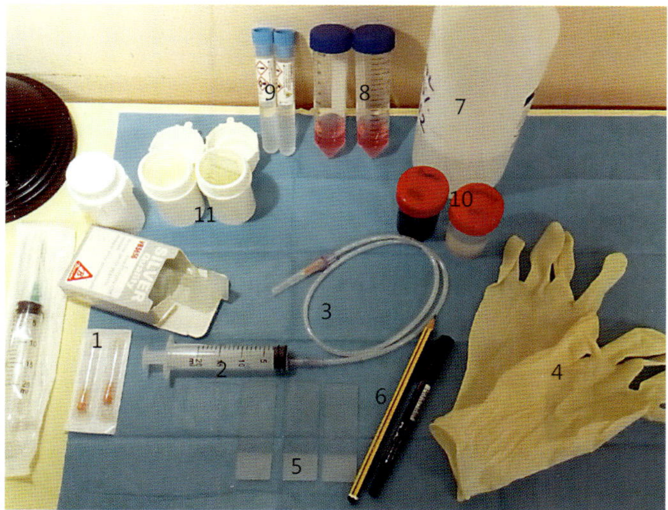

Fig. 1. Equipment to perform FNAC. Thin (25-G) sterile needles (1), sterile syringe (2) with flexible connector (3), gloves (4), glass slides with a rough end (5) on which the name of the patient can be written with a pencil (6), 95% alcohol to fix material for Pap staining (7), vials for liquid-based cytology (8) and cell block preparations (9), dyes for fast staining (10), and containers for the slides collected (11).

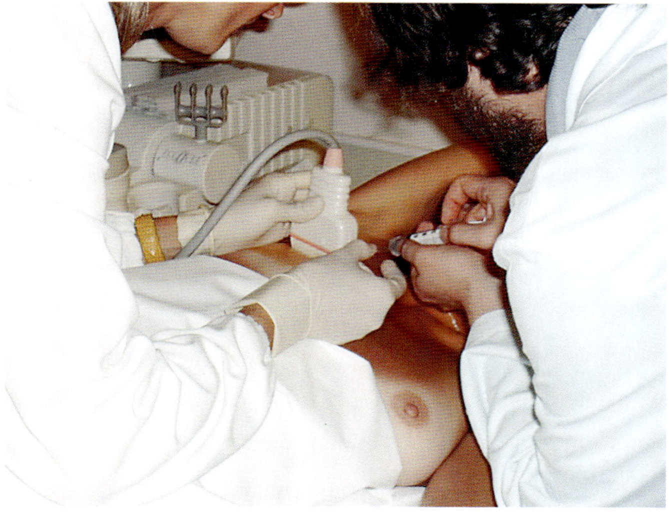

Fig. 2. FNA under ultrasound guidance using needle and syringe. Negative pressure is created in the syringe by pulling the piston up to 5–6 mL. The negative pressure should be maintained constant for 5–12 s, then the piston should be delicately released, and the needle withdrawn.

Following the recommendations of the National Cancer Institute sponsored conference [1996], the average number of FNAC passes recommended for adequate sampling of most breast lesions is 2–4, with no significant advantages of more passes. Lesions smaller than 1 cm do not require further passes after the third one. More passes could be useful only if the lesion is difficult to stabilize or penetrate, only scant material or a dry tap is obtained, the lesion is larger than 4 cm, or more material is needed for special studies.

Sampling Methods

Needle and Syringe (plus Syringe Holder): One Operator

This is the most widely used method for palpable lumps. After quick antisepsis of the skin above the lesion, the operator blocks the lump between the first two fingers of his or her left hand. Then, with the other hand, the operator rapidly inserts the needle attached to the syringe tip inside the mass. By pulling the piston, the operator creates a negative pressure of 5–6 mL inside the syringe and maintains it constant during the procedure (Fig. 2). The cytological material is collected by rotating the needle and moving it back and forth, always remaining inside the lump, for 5–12 s. After this time, the piston is delicately released, returning to its resting position, and only then the needle is rapidly retracted. The needle is separated from the syringe, which is partially filled with air and attached again to the needle. By gently pushing the piston, the collected material is expressed onto the slide to be spread.

The use of a syringe holder during this procedure renders the aspiration easier, but reduces the tactile perception of the lesion during the examination.

Needle, Syringe and Flexible Connector: Two Operators

In this procedure, the needle is attached to a flexible cannula or connector, which is in turn attached to the syringe (Fig. 3). After skin antisepsis, the first operator blocks the lesion and inserts the needle. Then, a second operator holding the syringe performs the aspiration by pulling the piston and creating a negative pressure of up to 10–18 mL. The cytological material is collected by rotating the needle, which remains always inside the lump, and moving it back and forth for 5–12 s. After this time, the second operator delicately releases the piston, and the first operator rapidly retracts the needle. Syringe, connector, and needle are quickly disassembled, and the syringe, partially filled with air, is used to push the collected material from the needle onto the slide.

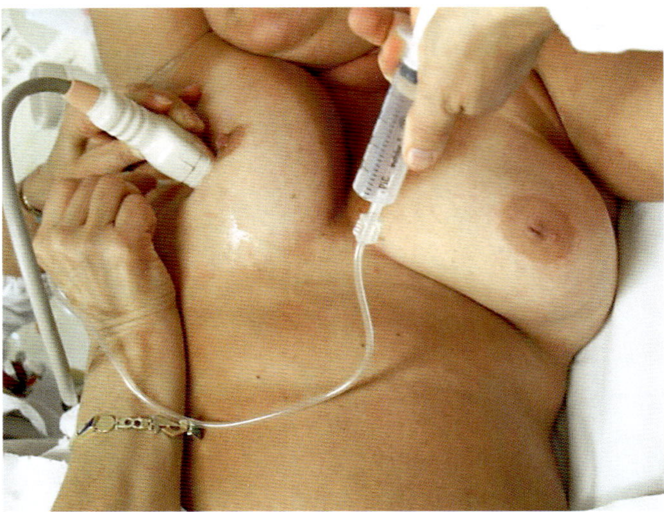

Fig. 3. FNA with needle, syringe, and connector. The aspiration is performed as in the method described in Figure 2, but the flexible connector minimizes the traumatic effect on cells, and the quality of the sample is generally better. Drawback: 2 operators are needed to obtain the aspirate.

This is the best aspiration method, because a flexible connector between needle and syringe minimizes the traumatic effect on the patient and aspirated cells, but it requires the presence of two skilled operators. In the lucky event of a strict collaboration between radiologist and cytopathologist, the radiologist should be the first operator, guiding the penetration of the needle right inside the lesion using ultrasound, while the cytopathologist should hold the syringe, perform the aspiration, place the material on the slide, and spread the aspirate.

Needle Only: One Operator

Cells may be collected in the needle by capillarity without the need of aspiration, even if this requires more experience than the other methods to obtain sufficient material [Zajdela et al., 1987]. Using this method, after skin antisepsis, the mass is blocked between the first two fingers of the left hand, and the right hand is used to insert the needle. The cytological material is collected by rotating the needle, which remains always inside the lump, and moving it back and forth. These movements disrupt the tissue and cause the cells to go up into the lumen of the needle. When the material becomes visible at the mouth of the needle, it is retracted. A syringe partially filled with air is used to delicately push the material onto the slide to be spread.

This method has the advantage of enhancing fingertip sensitivity and needle control and reducing the risk of blood contamination. Switching to another technique is recommended if the lesion is fibrous or yields limited cellular material.

Spreading Methods

The material collected by aspiration is deposited on the surface of one or more glass slides and has to be correctly spread to allow a good reading and interpretation of slides. The aim of this procedure is to obtain a thin, even layer of cells without clots or crushing artifacts. Make sure to have an adequate number of clean glass slides already prepared available with the name and/or identification number of the patient before starting the aspiration in order to minimize the time between cell withdrawal and spreading to reduce coagulation and drying artifacts.

To drop the material on the glass slide, bring the needle tip to the slide, taking care to turn the notch downward, and let 1–2 drops fall 1–2 cm below the rough end of the slide by delicately pushing the syringe piston (Fig. 4). For the spreading, there are two methods that are widely used and recommended for different types of material. The "one-step method" is preferred for scant and dense material, like the one taken from the majority of breast solid masses. The "two-step method" is used mostly for liquid and hemorrhagic material.

One-Step Method

Spread the material on the slide by holding it with one hand and putting the flat surface of another glass slide over the material. Then move it smoothly, gently, and swiftly to the other end of the slide by applying light pressure. This spreading must be performed with a single, unidirectional, and fluid movement, with a constant pressure sufficient to flatten the material in a single layer on the glass slide but trying to avoid cell crushing (Fig. 5). Crushed nuclei with smudgy chromatin and elongated erythrocytes on microscopic evaluation indicate a smear made with too much force. Some cytopathologists perform this type of smear by holding the spreader slide perpendicular to the other, while others prefer to have the slides parallel to each other.

Two-Step Method

Bring the end of the spreader slide in contact with the fluid material on the other slide with an angle of 45° between them. Then, pull the spreader slide toward the rough edge of the specimen slide carrying the fluid and suspended par-

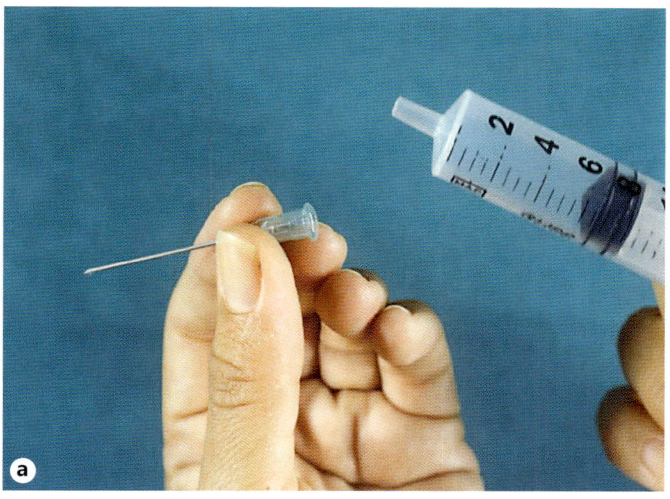

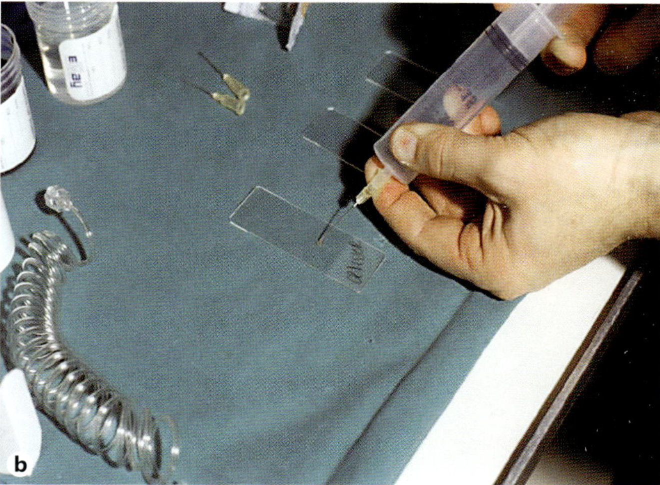

Fig. 4. Expelling of the aspirate on the glass slide. Immediately after the extraction of the needle, it is separated from the syringe (or from the connector). The syringe is partially filled with air and reconnected to the needle (**a**). Then, by applying light pressure on the piston, the material is gently expelled (not sprayed) on the glass slide (**b**).

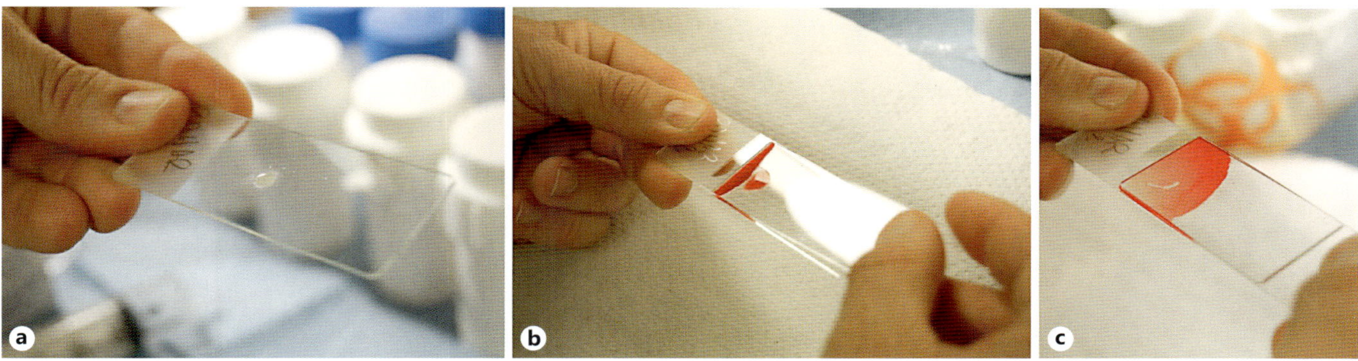

Fig. 5. Spreading. **a–c** Spreading is performed by putting the flat surface of another glass slide over the material and moving it smoothly, gently, and swiftly to the other end of the slide by applying gentle pressure. This spreading must be performed with a single, unidirectional movement, and with a constant, but not excessive, pressure.

ticles. Once there, change the direction of the spreading, bringing the material to the middle of the slide, where the tissue particles remain concentrated. Pull away the spreader slide from the other one and begin a second spreading, like the one-step method, beginning in the middle of the slide.

Once spread, slides planned for Papanicolaou staining must immediately be placed into a vial filled with 95% ethanol in order that the aspirated material is totally submerged in the alcohol solution. The ones planned for May-Grünwald-Giemsa (MGG) staining are left to dry in the open air.

Complications

FNAC is considered one of the safest invasive diagnostic procedures. Complications are rare and almost never severe. The most frequent complication is hematoma formation at the puncture site, which occurs in 3–5% of patients, especially in those taking anticoagulants. Nevertheless, the risk of a severe hemorrhage after FNAC is low enough to not require anticoagulant discontinuation before the examination. Hematoma formation may be prevented by the application of pressure on the sampling site immediately after performing FNAC. The nurse assisting in the procedure

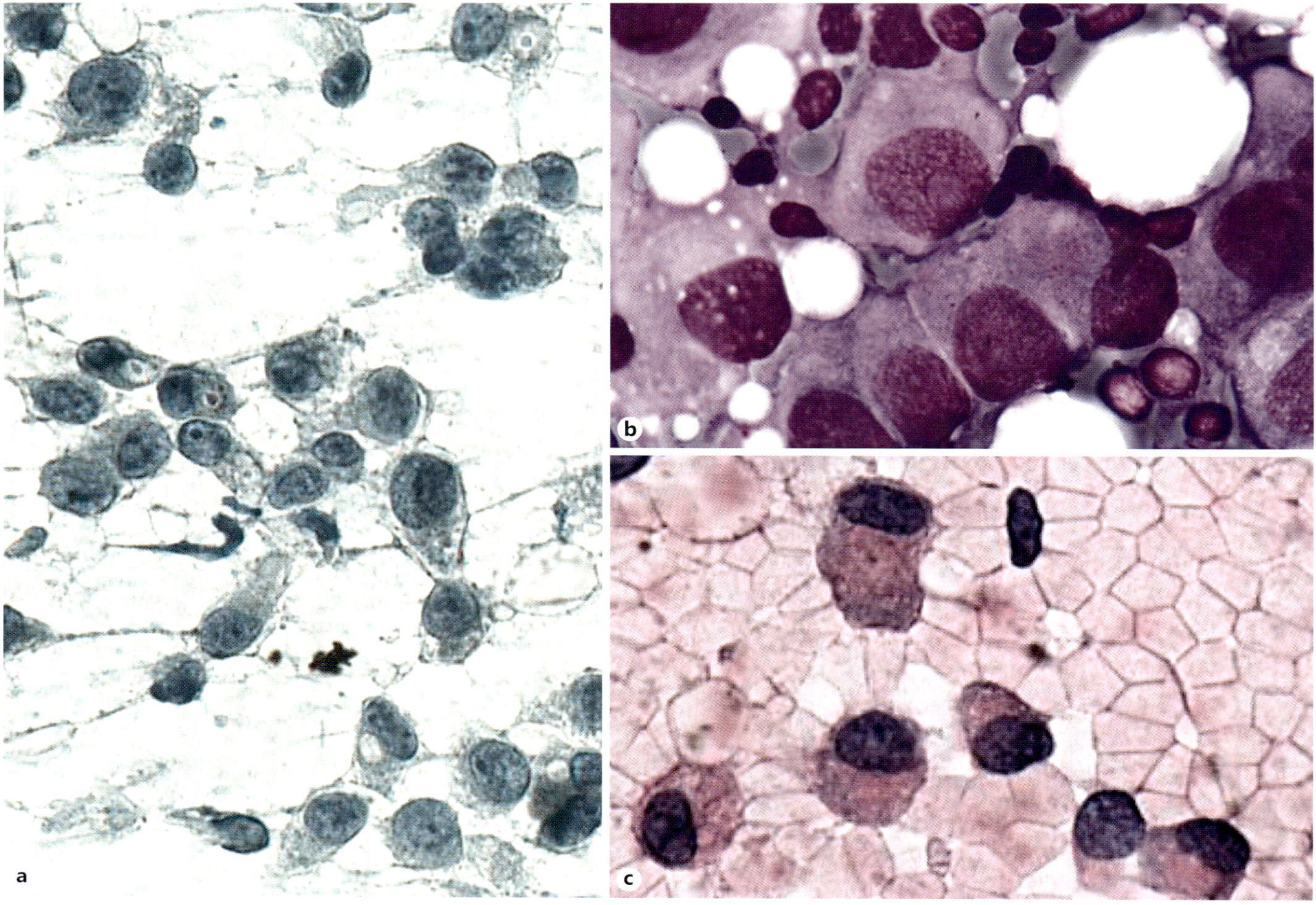

Fig. 6. Types of staining used in cytology. Papanicolaou staining (**a**) allows a better evaluation of nuclear chromatin compared with May-Grünwald-Giemsa (MGG) (**b**) but requires immediate fixation in alcohol. MGG stain is performed on air-dried material and is preferred for an accurate evaluation of the cytoplasm and background. Cells generally appear larger than they are stained with Papanicolaou. H&E has similar advantages and disadvantages as Papanicolaou staining, but it is less used in cytology (**c**).

usually first takes care of it and then asks the patient to press the site with a dry swab or an ice pack for 5–10 min.

Discomfort during and after the procedure is common, but pain is typically minimal and does not require the administration of local anesthetics, which may be more painful than the biopsy itself. However, anesthetics should be administered on patient request since pain is an extremely subjective feeling. Fully explaining the procedure can help to minimize patient discomfort during the examination [Boinon et al., 2017]. Areas most frequently reported as painful during the procedure are those adjacent to the nipple. Any pain after FNAC can be relieved with nonprescription analgesics like paracetamol.

Infection is rare; it can be avoided by careful skin cleansing and using sterile disposable items and equipment. When it occurs, it is generally ascribed to cutaneous bacterial flora and may require the administration of antibiotics.

Pneumothorax is a recognized complication, and incidence rates reported in the literature range from 0.01 to 3% [Bates et al., 2002]. Risk factors are deep breast lumps, thin body build, and breath holding during the procedure. The complication has been associated with FNA in any of the four quadrants of the breast but especially with aspiration in the outer-upper quadrant. In 50–80% of cases, no specific treatment is needed; the remainder require insertion of a chest drain. The risk of pneumothorax can be lessened by

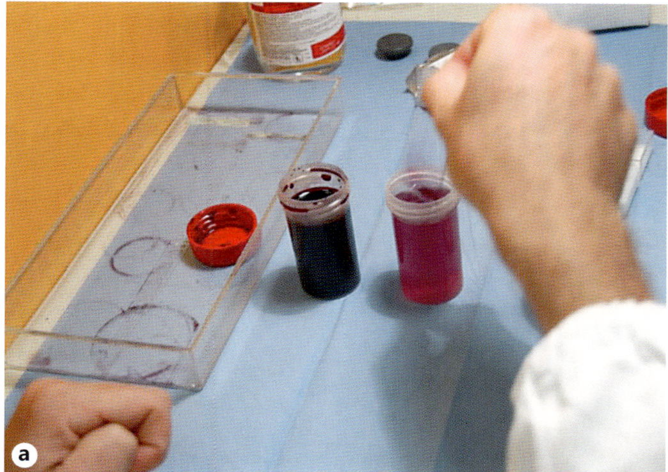

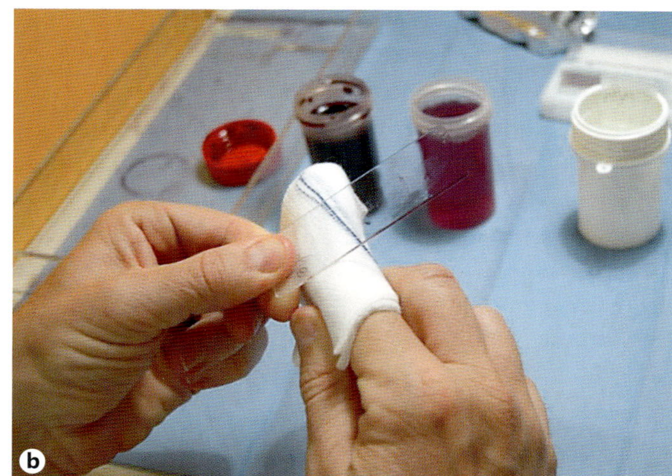

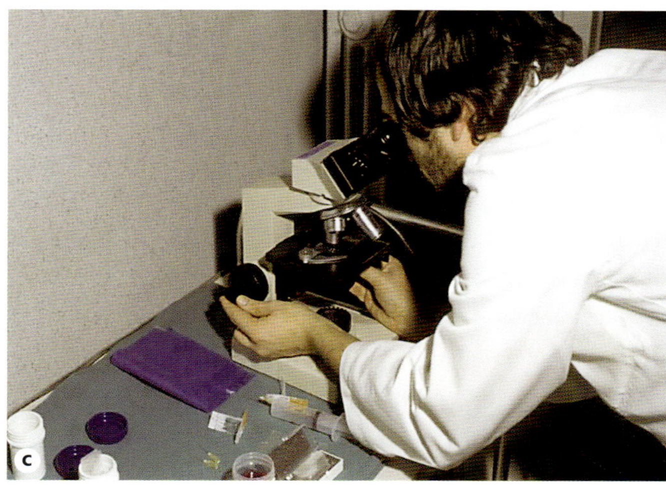

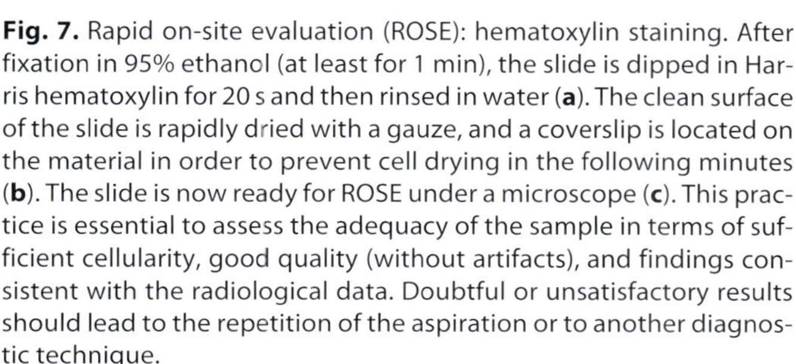

Fig. 7. Rapid on-site evaluation (ROSE): hematoxylin staining. After fixation in 95% ethanol (at least for 1 min), the slide is dipped in Harris hematoxylin for 20 s and then rinsed in water (**a**). The clean surface of the slide is rapidly dried with a gauze, and a coverslip is located on the material in order to prevent cell drying in the following minutes (**b**). The slide is now ready for ROSE under a microscope (**c**). This practice is essential to assess the adequacy of the sample in terms of sufficient cellularity, good quality (without artifacts), and findings consistent with the radiological data. Doubtful or unsatisfactory results should lead to the repetition of the aspiration or to another diagnostic technique.

the technique: the patient should breathe normally, and the needle should be inserted into the mass parallel rather than perpendicular to the chest wall whenever possible, especially in thin patients with small breasts. Furthermore, it is advisable that patients with deep, centrally located, and small or nonpalpable lesions have their FNAC under ultrasound guidance [Liao et al., 2004].

Staining Methods

Cytological slides may be stained with Papanicolaou, MGG, or hematoxylin and eosin (H&E) (Fig. 6). Whether to use a staining method or another is mainly a matter of habits. Papanicolaou staining was first developed for cervicovaginal cytology and is currently used for all the exfoliative cytology, but it can be used in any field; it is generally preferred by cytopathologists who base their diagnoses on the accurate evaluation of nuclear chromatin, which is better visualized with Pap staining. MGG was first developed by hematologists and is more frequently used in most aspiration cytology. Since these two types of staining are often complementary, an expert cytopathologist should be able to interpret smears stained with both methods correctly. H&E is primarily a staining for histological samples, but some pathologists use it also in cytology.

Rapid On-Site Evaluation

ROSE of cytological specimens allows immediate assessment of the cellular content and adequacy of FNAC smears and the identification of those that are clearly positive. Based on this information, the operator decides whether or not additional samples or a repetition of the procedure are needed, which also affects costs in this cost-conscious age [Nasuti et al., 2002; Delaloge et al., 2016]. If repeat FNAC are still inadequate, the mass should be reevaluated by the radiologist and, if suspicion persists, another diagnostic technique should be applied, such as CNB. The immediate identification of malignant lesions at ROSE allows the clinicians to accelerate the diagnostic assessment and therapeutic management of the patient, potentially reducing the time between preoperative examinations and treatment.

ROSE methodology varies, especially regarding the type of stain used [Silverman et al., 1990; Yang and Alvarez, 1995; Thierry et al., 2012]. While the definitive staining is normally performed by cytotechnologists in the laboratory, the rapid ones are performed directly in the clinic, so the operator performing the FNAC, whoever it is, should know the procedure to obtain a well-stained slide.

The most commonly used staining is Diff-Quik, which is a modified MGG staining that requires only 40 s to be set up. Similar to all the slides planned to be stained with MGG, those to be stained with Diff-Quik must be air dried. This staining method is performed as follows:

- Greenish-blue QuickLink III fixative (methanol): dip the slide in the greenish-blue methanol fixative 20 times.
- Dark-orange QuickLink solution I (sodium azide): dip the slide in the dark-orange sodium azide solution 20 times.
- Dark-blue QuickLink solution II (hematoxylin): dip the slide in the dark-blue hematoxylin solution 20 times.
- Water: dip the slide in water 20 times to rinse it

After the slide has been stained and air dried again, it is ready to be viewed under a microscope. Slides stained in this way must not be decolored or restained.

Another common way to obtain rapidly stained smears is to use just hematoxylin after prefixation in 95% ethanol. The slide is dipped in a hyperconcentrated hematoxylin solution (Harris hematoxylin) for 20 s and then rinsed in water. After placing a coverslip on the slide and drying the excess water with a gauze, the sample is ready to be viewed under a microscope (Fig. 7). This rapid staining allows a quick evaluation of the nuclei, which is sufficient to assess sample adequacy and to identify many malignant lesions. The slides stained in this way may be decolored and restained with Papanicolaou, so this is the preferred rapid staining for cytopathologists who are more accustomed to the Papanicolaou stain.

References

Bates T, Davidson T, Mansel RE: Litigation for pneumothorax as a complication of fine needle aspiration of the breast. Br J Surg 2002;89:134–137.

Boinon D, Dauchy S, Charles C, Fasse L, Cano A, Balleyguier C, Mazouni C, Caron H, Vielh P, Delaloge S: Patient satisfaction with a rapid diagnosis of suspicious breast lesions: association with distress and anxiety. Breast J 2017, DOI: 10.1111/tbj.12856. Epub ahead of print.

Delaloge S, Bonastre J, Borget I, Garbay JR, Fontenay R, Boinon D, Saghatchain M, Mathieu MC, Mazouni C, Rivera S, Uzan C, André F, Dromain C, Boyer B, Pistilli B, Azoulay S, Rimareix F, Bayou el-H, Sarfati B, Caron H, Ghouadni A, Leymarie N, Canale S, Mons M, Arfi-Rouche J, Arnedos M, Suciu V, Vielh P, Balleyguier C: The challenge of rapid diagnosis in oncology: diagnostic accuracy and cost analysis of a large-scale one-stop breast clinic. Eur J Cancer 2016;66:131–137.

Domanski AM, Monsef N, Domanski HA, Grabau D, Fernö M: Comparison of the oestrogen and progesterone receptor status in primary breast carcinomas as evaluated by immunohistochemistry and immunocytochemistry: a consecutive series of 267 patients. Cytopathology 2013;24:21–25.

Ferguson J, Chamberlain P, Cramer HM, Wu HH: ER, PR, and Her2 immunocytochemistry on cell-transferred cytologic smears of primary and metastatic breast carcinomas: a comparison study with formalin-fixed cell blocks and surgical biopsies. Diagn Cytopathol 2013;41:575–581.

Garbar C, Curé H: Fine-needle aspiration cytology can play a role in neoadjuvant chemotherapy in operable breast cancer. ISRN Oncol 2013;2013:935796.

Kocjan G, Bourgain C, Fassina A, Hagmar B, Herbert A, et al: The role of breast FNAC in diagnosis and clinical management: a survey of current practice. Cytopathology 2008;19:271–278.

Liao J, Davey DD, Warren G, Davis J, Moore AR, Samayoa LM: Ultrasound-guided fine-needle aspiration biopsy remains a valid approach in the evaluation of nonpalpable breast lesions. Diagn Cytopathol 2004;30:325–331.

Nasuti JF, Gupta PK, Baloch ZW: Diagnostic value and cost-effectiveness of on-site evaluation of fine-needle aspiration specimens: review of 5,688 cases. Diagn Cytopathol 2002;27:1–4.

National Cancer Institute sponsored conference. The uniform approach to breast fine-needle aspiration biopsy. Diagn Cytopathol 1997;16:295–311.

Silverman JF, Frable WJ: The use of the Diff-Quik stain in the immediate interpretation of fine-needle aspiration biopsies. Diagn Cytopathol 1990;6: 366–369.

Thierry R, Marie-Christine R, Mariele M, Richard B, Anca M: Modified technique of toluidine blue staining in rapid on-site evaluation. Diagn Cytopathol 2012;40:847–848.

Vural G, Hagmar B, Lilleng R: A one-year audit of fine needle aspiration cytology of breast lesions. Factors affecting adequacy and a review of delayed carcinoma diagnoses. Acta Cytol 1995;39:1233–1236.

Willems SM, van Deurzen CH, van Diest PJ: Diagnosis of breast lesions: fine-needle aspiration cytology or core needle biopsy? A review. J Clin Pathol 2012;65:287–292.

Yang GC, Alvarez II: Ultrafast Papanicolaou stain. An alternative preparation for fine needle aspiration cytology. Acta Cytol 1995;39:55–60.

Zagorianakou P, Fiaccavento S, Zagorianakou N, Makrydimas G, Stefanou D, Agnantis NJ: FNAC: its role, limitations and perspective in the preoperative diagnosis of breast cancer. Eur J Gynaecol Oncol 2005;26:240.

Zajdela A, Vielh P, Di Bonito L: Manuel et Atlas de Cytologie Mammaire. Piccin, 1995. ISBN: 88-299-1188-7.

Zajdela A, Zillhardt P, Voillemot N: Cytological diagnosis by fine needle sampling without aspiration. Cancer 1987;59:1201–1205.

Pinamonti M, Zanconati F: Breast Cytopathology. Assessing the Value of FNAC in the Diagnosis of Breast Lesions.
Monogr Clin Cytol. Basel, Karger, 2018, vol 24, pp 9–19 (DOI: 10.1159/000479763)

Principles of Interpretation

Clinical and Radiological Information

Dealing with breast lesions, cytopathologists should understand that they are not alone in the diagnostic process, but they are part of an ordered inquiry managed by a multidisciplinary team. Following is a brief list of relevant clinical information that we suggest to be collected by the operator during the aspiration session:

- Age of the patient
- Familiar history of breast cancer
- Previous breast surgery, radiation, or chemotherapy
- Eventual pregnant or lactating status
- Dimension of the lesion
- Onset and evolution of the lesion over the time
- Precise location of the lesion
- Clinical features of the lesion
- Mammographic and/or ultrasound features of the lesion

Being provided with this information might be fundamental to correctly interpret the smear. For example, knowing that a certain lesion has a stellate aspect and is highly suspicious on the mammogram may focus the attention of the cytopathologist to the slight cytological atypia and possibly recognize a well-differentiated carcinoma that could otherwise be misdiagnosed as a benign lesion. Likewise, being aware of the pregnancy status of the patient should lead the cytopathologist to reconsider his or her conclusions about a highly proliferative lesion.

FNAC results should always be interpreted in the context of the so-called triple test [Kline et al., 1999], which comprises the following components:

1 Clinical breast examination and medical history
2 Imaging – mammography and/or ultrasound
3 Nonexcisional biopsy – FNAC and/or core needle biopsy

The triple test is positive if any of the 3 components is positive, and negative if all the components are negative. The triple test has a sensitivity of 99.6% and a specificity of 93% [Irwig and Macaskill, 1997]. When the triple test is concordant, final treatment can be ensued safely. In nonconcordant cases, FNAC stands as the single most important investigation. However, due to its possible false-negative results, other components of the triple test need to be employed to enhance its efficacy and diagnostic yield [Ahmed et al., 2007]. Accurate interpretation requires a close working relationship between the managing clinician, the radiologist, and the pathologist. When a discrepancy between the 3 components occurs, further workup is needed. This could include the clinical and/or radiological revaluation of the case or a new pathological investigation, which could be obtained through core or excision biopsy.

Clinical Features of Breast Lesions

Breast lesions may present at any age with different symptoms due to their dimensions, location, consistency, and functional characteristics. The main symptoms of breast lesions include a palpable mass, pain, unusual nipple discharge, and eventually reddening or change in the quality of the skin above. When a palpable mass is present, its location should be described as being in 1 of 4 quadrants of the breast and/or by referring to the clock hours, from the point of view of the examiner, and by specifying the distance from the nipple in order to enable a comparison with subsequent evaluations of the same mass and to guide subsequent diagnostic and therapeutic operations. Clinical features of the mass, such as shape, borders, consistency, and mobility, must be carefully evaluated.

To proceed with the clinical evaluation of a breast mass, the patient's breast should be uncovered (i.e., shirt and bra removed), and the patient possibly lying flat on a table. The arm of the side to be examined should be placed behind the head to expose the breast completely and allow easy access of the ipsilateral axilla. In this position, it is possible to perform ultrasound and FNAC, eventually asking the patient to position herself on the side opposite to the one to be examined to make lateral lesions easier to reach.

Normal breasts have a lumpy consistency, created by the mix of glandular, fibrous, and adipose tissue. Masses of concern tend to have the following characteristics: they are different from the rest of the breast tissue and firm, and borders are irregular and hard to define. Masses are fixed/stuck to adjacent tissue and increase in size over time. Breast density decreases with age, so it is relatively easier to identify masses in older patients.

Malignant lesions have a general tendency to infiltrate the surrounding tissue, evoking a desmoplastic stromal reaction that may cause retraction and inversion of the nipple if the lesion is located near the areolar region.

Despite the frequent involvement of the large duct system, the abnormal nipple discharge is generally not considered as a classical symptom of breast carcinoma, being more typical of papillary lesions. These lesions may present with a unilateral, intermittent, serous, or bloody secretion from the nipple. The examiner, through a gentle pressure in the areolar area, may provoke the nipple discharge and then collect the material and spread it on a glass slide in order to be examined under a microscope. This could help in obtaining useful cytological material and eventually lead to a diagnosis without any invasive procedure.

Skin redness, pain, and eventually a purulent discharge from the nipple are the classical symptoms of infective and inflammatory breast lesions. Nevertheless, breast cancer might be associated with inflammation, especially in the dramatic presentation of inflammatory breast carcinoma or *mastitis carcinomatosa*. In this rare occurrence, the breast appears completely flushed, hot, painful, and swollen, and often a mass cannot be identified clinically and radiologically due to the massive edema and inflammation of the breast tissue. Distinguishing advanced cancer from a purely inflammatory process could be challenging, as both FNAC and core needle biopsies cannot be performed in the absence of a clearly identifiable target. Since inflammatory breast carcinoma is caused by the extensive involvement and obstruction of dermal lymph vessels by breast cancer, skin biopsies, performed generally in the periareolar region, might help to get valuable diagnostic material and guide the subsequent therapeutic choices.

In the following chapters, the clinical features of each breast lesion will be briefly described.

Possible Radiological Interpretations

Mammography may be able to detect breast cancer before symptoms develop. Although this is not universally true for all breast lesions, its usefulness as a diagnostic tool is undisputed, and it is largely used all over the world to detect and characterize breast lesions, both in symptomatic and nonsymptomatic women. Being a highly sensitive technique, it is universally accepted as the first-line diagnostic tool in population-based screening programs.

The method makes use of X-rays to study the breast parenchyma and identify calcifications, lumps, or changes in the fibrous architecture of the breast (Fig. 1). The accuracy of mammography is related to breast density, being higher in older women with a greater fat component in the breast structure.

Ultrasound has traditionally been used as a complementary tool to improve the specificity of clinical and mammographic findings. It is not only able to distinguish solid from liquid lesions, it can also highlight a number of features that allow a highly accurate diagnosis of breast lesions in expert hands using modern ultrasound equipment. Masses are characterized according to their shape, orientation, margins, echo pattern, posterior acoustic features, surrounding tissue features, and the presence of calcifications.

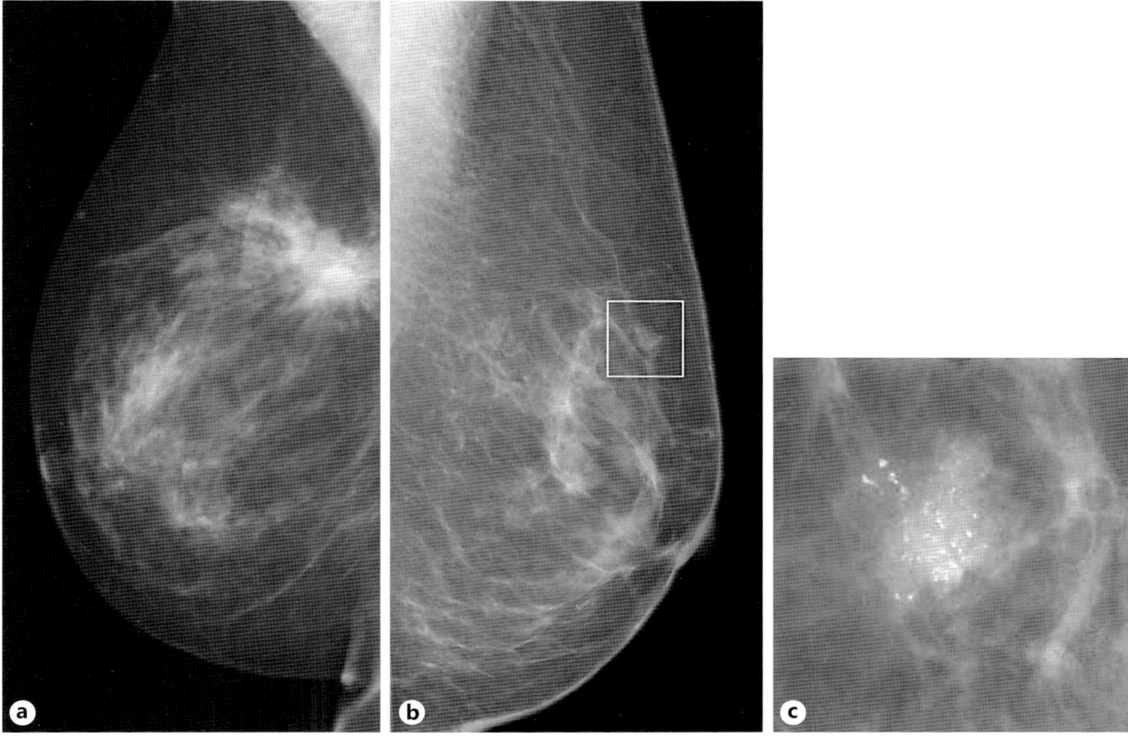

Fig. 1. Mammography. Breast cancer might be visualized by mammography as an irregular opacity against radiotransparent adipose tissue (**a**) or due to the presence of microcalcifications (**b**). **c** Higher magnification of the rectangle shown in **b**.

Generally, solid benign lesions, such as fibroadenomas, appear as well-circumscribed, oval or round-shaped, hypoechoic masses, typically oriented parallel to the skin, while invasive ductal carcinomas can have an irregular shape, spiculated margins, and acoustic shadowing, a peculiar phenomenon unique to sonography, indicating the desmoplastic response of the tissue (Fig. 2) [Candelaria et al., 2013].

In order to standardize the radiological reporting, improving the communication between medical professionals, the American College of Radiology (ACR) designed the BI-RADS (Breast Imaging-Reporting and Data System) lexicon, which expresses the risk of malignancy of a breast lesion on a scale from 0 to 5.

BI-RADS
0 Examination incomplete or not performed
1 Negative examination, no lesion detected
2 Benign findings
3 Undetermined, probably benign
4 Suspicious for malignancy
5 Highly suggestive of malignancy

BI-RADS is a quality assurance tool originally designed for use with mammography but also adopted for ultrasound and magnetic resonance imaging. Some experts believe that the single BI-RADS 4 classification does not adequately communicate the risk of cancer to doctors and recommend the following subclassification scheme [Sanders et al., 2010]:
4A Low suspicion for malignancy
4B Intermediate suspicion of malignancy
4C Moderate concern, but not classic for malignancy

Additionally to the BI-RADS score, mammography reports often include a second score referring to the breast composition and density [D'Orsi et al., 2013]:
A The breasts are almost entirely fatty
B There are scattered areas of fibroglandular density
C The breasts are heterogeneously dense, which may obscure small masses
D The breasts are extremely dense, which lowers the sensitivity of mammography

According to the guidelines from the National Cancer Institute sponsored conference [1997], lesions that may be subjected to nonexcisional diagnostic biopsy (FNAC or core

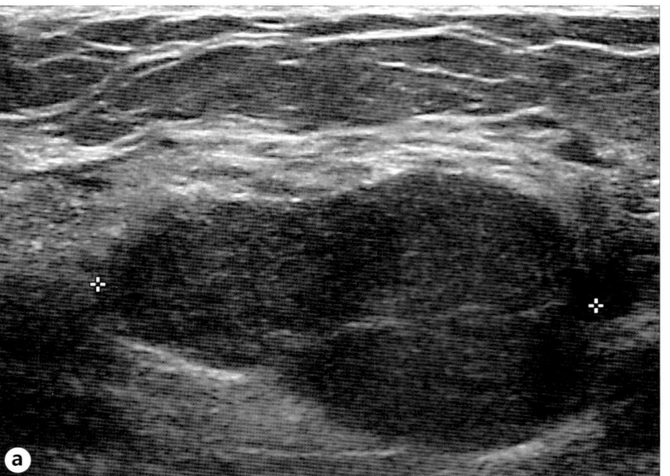

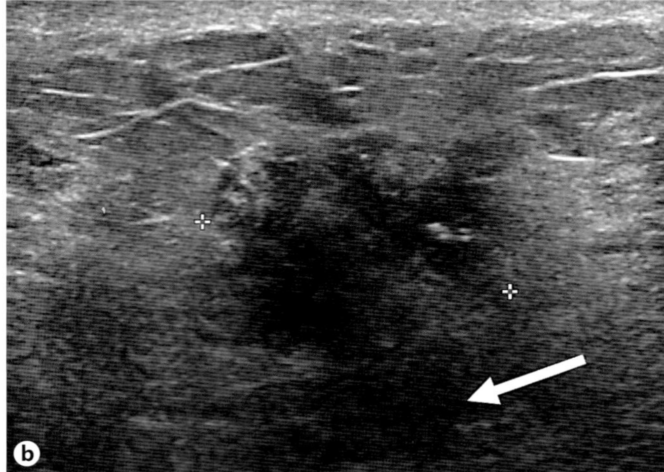

Fig. 2. Breast ultrasound. Solid lumps appear hypoechoic (dark gray) compared to the surrounding hyperechoic (light gray) adipose parenchyma. Benign lesions such as fibroadenomas are generally oval shaped, with distinct round borders and a long axis parallel to the skin (**a**). Breast carcinomas frequently show irregular margins and posterior acoustic shadowing (arrow) (**b**).

needle biopsy) include those that are suspicious (BI-RADS 4) or highly suggestive of malignancy (BI-RADS 5), and some of the ones at low risk of malignancy (BI-RADS 3) for which the recommended follow-up with imaging is not feasible or accepted by the patient.

Major Morphological Criteria

Differently from exfoliative cytology, FNAC sample cells come from a specific part of the organ, which was previously identified as suspicious or pathological by clinical or radiological examination. Thus, if the sampling has been correctly performed, all the cells in the smear come from that mass and have to be examined carefully. The analysis starts at low magnification (×5 and ×10 lens) to rapidly assess the adequacy of the sample and get an idea of the cellular yield and the aggregation status of the cells. At this point, increasing the magnification, the analysis passes to the characteristics of the nuclei and the cytoplasm of cells.

While viewing the smear, the cytopathologist takes several morphological features into account that should be considered together in order to reach a correct diagnosis. Before describing the specific morphological characteristics of the single breast lesions in detail, we find it useful to focus on the characteristics that should be carefully considered and the general criteria to be able to distinguish benign from malignant lesions. It is important to stress that the concept of "atypia," which is frequently advocated by many cytopathologists, is largely subjective, and there are no well-defined criteria to definitely categorize findings of atypia in breast cytology [Lim et al., 2004].

Following is a brief checklist of the most important morphological criteria to be considered:

- Cellularity
- Size and shape of cellular aggregates
- Cohesiveness of aggregates
- Presence of myoepithelial cells
- Bare nuclei
- Single cells with intact cytoplasm
- Nature of background
- Nuclear size, shape, and membrane
- Nuclear chromatin
- Nucleoli: presence, number, and quality
- Nuclear/cytoplasmic ratio
- Color and size of the cytoplasm
- Cellular pleomorphism
- Mitoses

The value attributed to the single aspects varies between different pathologists. A large study assessing reproducibility in many Indian cytology centers tried to determine the cytopathologists' perception of the various morphological aspects. The most significant feature turned out to be the nuclear chromatin pattern, while the less significant ones were the nature of the background and the color and size of the cytoplasm (still considered by most as "moderately sig-

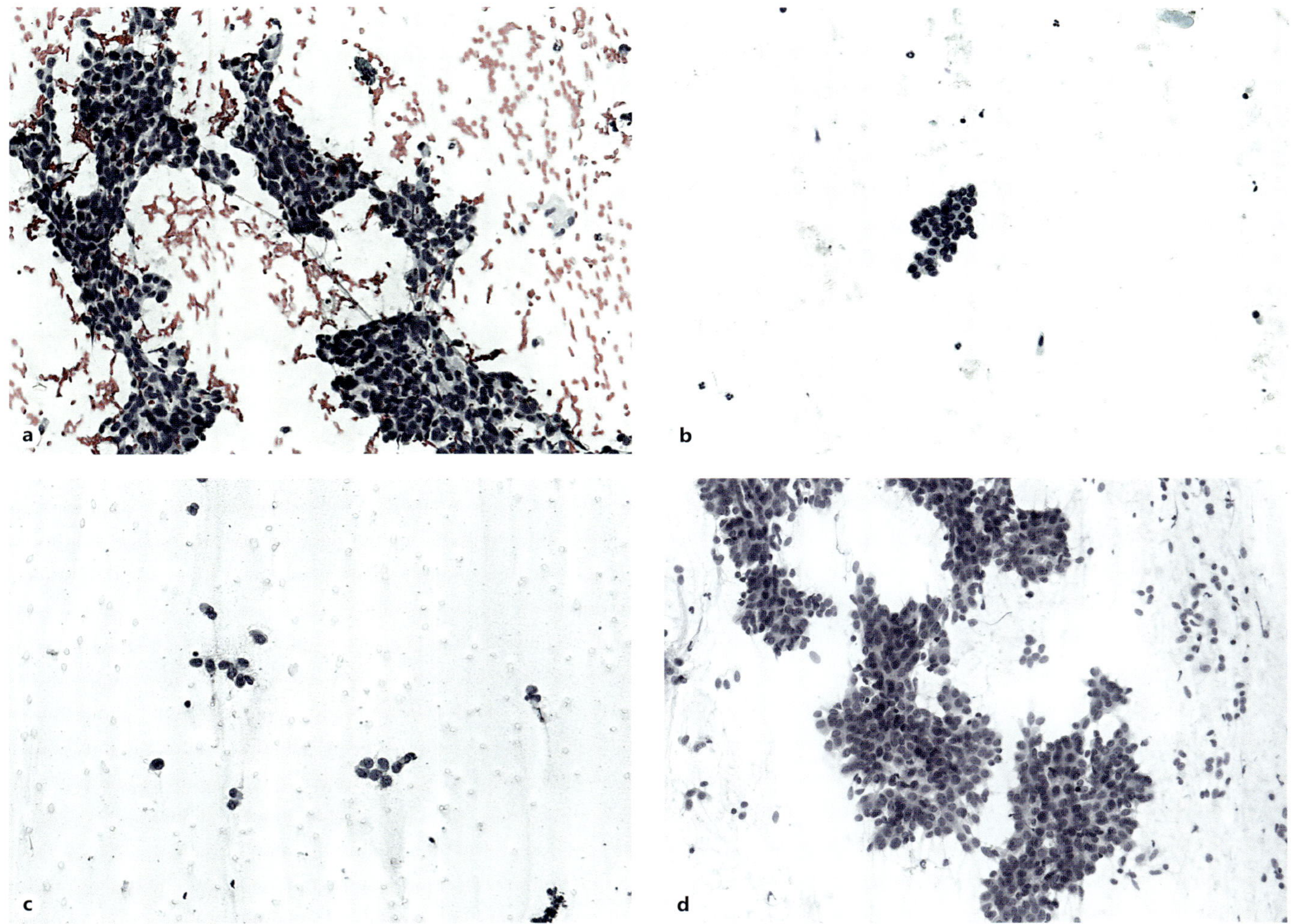

Fig. 3. Smear cellularity. Aspirates from invasive ductal carcinomas typically show moderate to high cellularity (**a**) compared to benign lesions (**b**). On the other hand, highly sclerotic malignant lesions and lobular carcinomas usually display very scant cellularity (**c**), and some benign lesions, such as juvenile fibroadenomas, may produce highly cellular smears (**d**). Papanicolaou. Intermediate power.

nificant"). The perception about the features showed a converging trend with increasing experience [Garud, 2012].

In our opinion, there is not a single feature that is more important than one of the others, and the whole set of cytological characteristics must be properly assessed and weighed to reach a correct diagnosis.

Cellularity

Aspirates from malignant lesions frequently show moderate or abundant cellularity. On the other hand, carcinomas with marked desmoplastic reaction or those with a low density of cancer cells produce poorly cellular smears, and results are frequently inadequate, while some benign lesions such as some juvenile fibroadenomas and intraductal papillomas provide highly cellular smears (Fig. 3).

Cellular Aggregates

Most benign lesions produce large and cohesive single-layer sheets of epithelial cells with neat borders and sometimes finger-like ends, while cellular aggregates aspirated from many carcinomas tend to be 3-dimensional and very inhomogeneous, with coexistence of large and small clusters, irregular shapes, and a greater tendency to lose cohesion (Fig. 4). However, some benign lesions such as sclerosing adenosis and intraductal papillomas are characterized by the presence of many small cellular clusters and isolated epithelial cells.

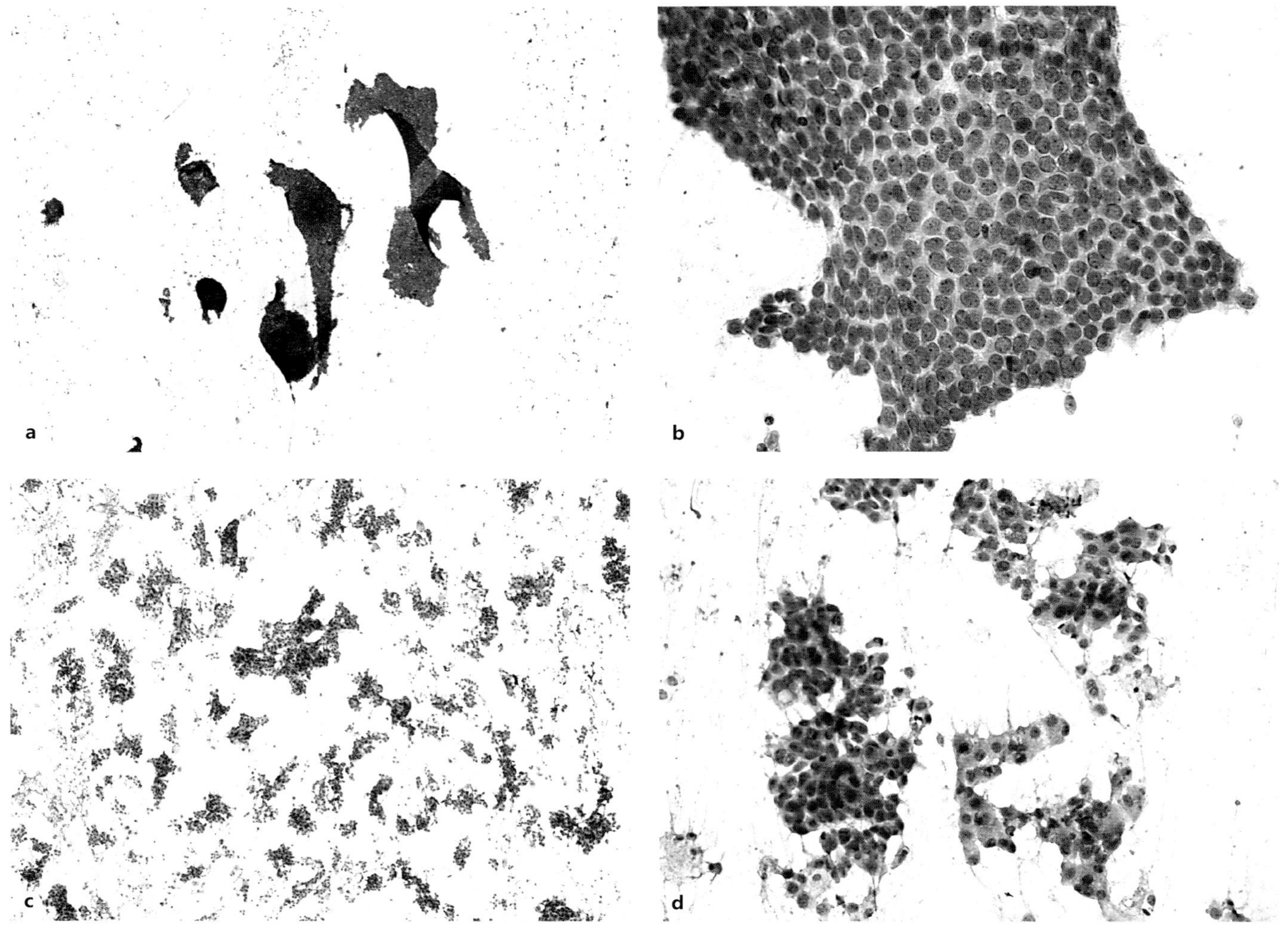

Fig. 4. Cellular aggregates. Benign lesions usually show large, cohesive monolayer sheets of uniformly distributed ductal cells with neat borders (**a**, **b**), while cellular cluster aspirations of an invasive carcinoma are frequently irregular in size and shape, have a disordered distribution of the nuclei, and a greater tendency to lose cell-to-cell cohesion (**c**, **d**). Papanicolaou. **a**, **c** Scanning magnification. **b**, **d** Intermediate power.

Myoepithelial Cells and Bare Nuclei

The absence of myoepithelial cells and bare nuclei [described in Chapter 3, this vol., pp. 20–24] is one of the most used criteria to identify an invasive (malignant) lesion. Tubular carcinomas and some low-grade ductal carcinomas are exceptions to this rule, since a few myoepithelial cells may still be found despite the stromal invasion. Conversely, benign apocrine lesions frequently lack myoepithelial cells. Bare nuclei, as a sign of benignity, must be carefully examined since some carcinomas display a population of "naked" tumor cell nuclei. Usually, they have obvious malignant features, but some may be ovoid and, therefore, mistaken for bipolar nuclei.

Nuclear Features

Most malignant cells are easily recognized for their nuclear features: carcinoma cell nuclei are usually larger than those of normal ductal cells and have significant differences in size and shape between each other; nuclear chromatin tends to be coarse, clumped, and irregularly distributed, and nuclear membranes show indentations, folds, grooves, and clefts (Fig. 5). These nuclear features are more evident in high-grade carcinomas, while they tend to show nuances in well-differentiated tumors, which frequently show a certain degree of monomorphism. Malignant cell nuclei may show a variable tendency to rupture under the physical pressure of being smeared. This is not true for all carcinomas, but the

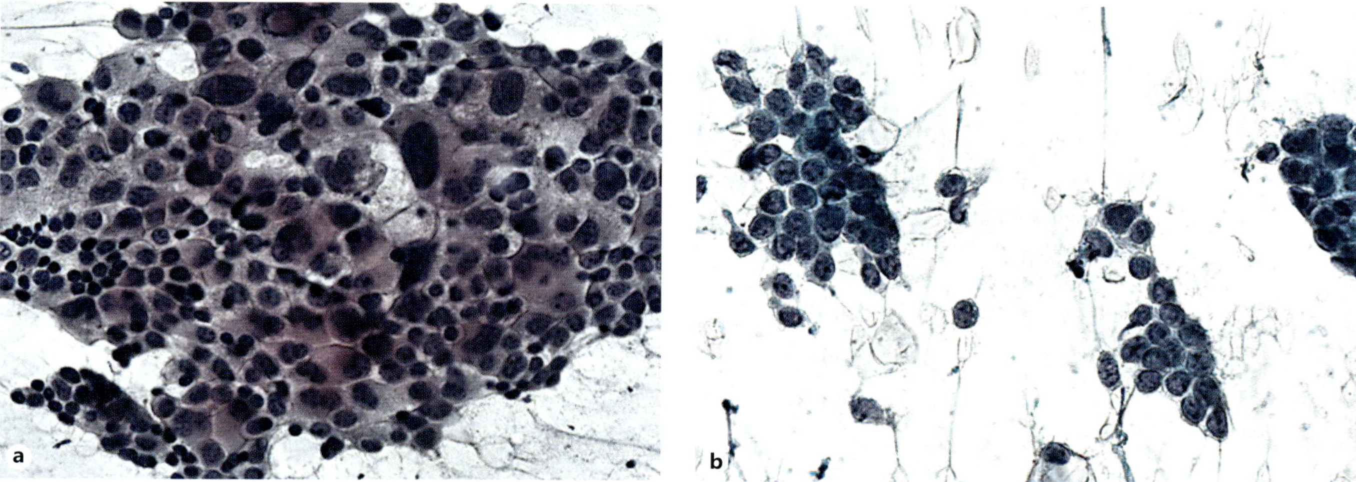

Fig. 5. Nuclear features. High-grade carcinomas show important variation in nuclear size and shape; nuclear contours may be irregular and chromatin frequently shows clumps, folds, and pseudo-inclusions (**a**). Conversely, cells of low-grade carcinomas are often rather monomorphic (**b**). Papanicolaou. High power.

presence of numerous crushing phenomena may suggest the presence of a poorly differentiated neoplasm (Fig. 6).

Nuclear morphometry (accurate evaluation of nuclear size, shape, and nuclear membrane irregularities) is also used to distinguish benign breast lesions from borderline lesions, such as atypical ductal hyperplasia, even though alterations are less pronounced than in most carcinomas [Kashyap et al., 2017]. Nuclear characteristics are generally more marked in Papanicolaou-stained preparations.

Nucleoli

A single, delicate nucleolus can be present in normal ductal cells, but prominent or multiple nucleoli represent a suspicious item. Many grade 2 or 3 carcinomas show prominent nucleoli, indicating increased cellular activity, but nucleoli alone are not sufficient to direct the diagnosis towards malignancy, since other conditions of increased ductal cell activity may produce equally large nucleoli. This is the case in breast changes during pregnancy and lactation, and some benign proliferative conditions, including fibroadenomas. Thus, they should be considered together with the nuclear chromatin features.

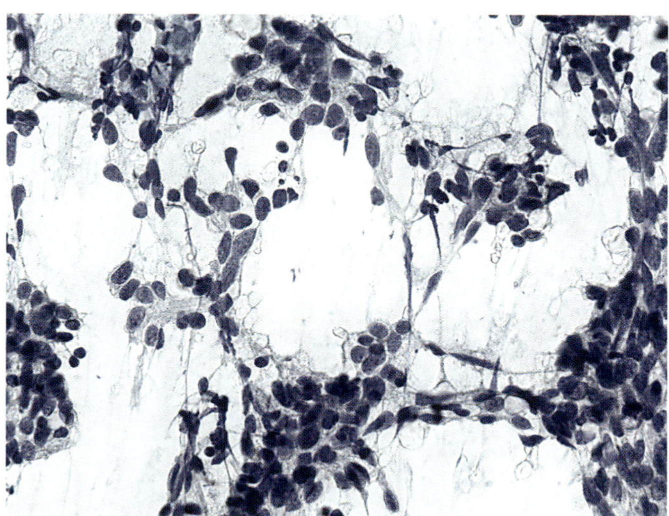

Fig. 6. High-grade carcinoma. Cells in the sample are poorly cohesive and irregularly distributed and have round, oval, elongated, or angulated shapes. Many crush artifacts are present due to extreme nuclear fragility. Papanicolaou. High power.

Nuclear/Cytoplasmic Ratio and Cytoplasmic Features

Dealing with breast lesions, the nuclear/cytoplasmic ratio is less important than in other cytology application fields, since the cytoplasm is typically scant in benign ductal cells and may be abundant in some ductal carcinomas. Multiple small, eosinophilic granules are present in the cytoplasm of cells with an apocrine differentiation, whether benign or malignant, and vacuoles or intracytoplasmic lumina can occasionally be seen in both lobular and ductal carcinoma cells as well as in some benign epithelial cells.

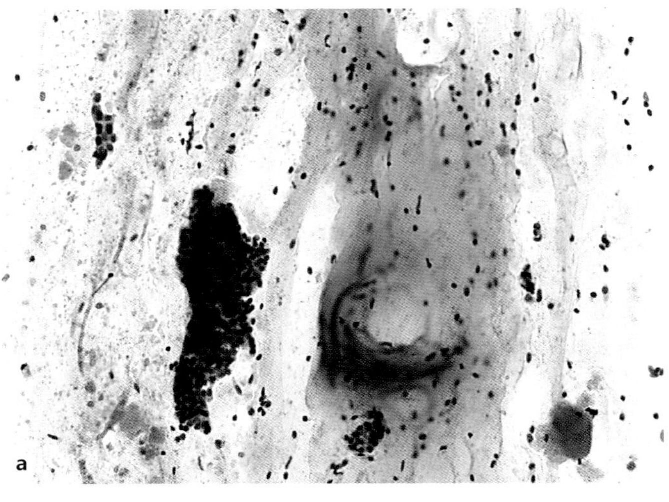

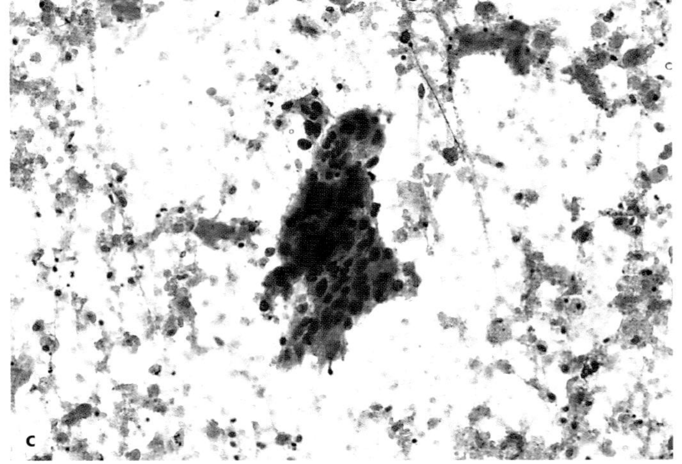

Fig. 7. Background. The background of the smear gives sometimes important additional information that may be useful to correctly interpret the aspirate together with the main cytological features. A myxoid background in a cellular and "benign-looking" smear may orient towards a diagnosis of fibroadenoma (**a**), but similar amorphous material is the key feature for the diagnosis of mucinous carcinoma in the presence of atypical cells (**b**). A highly necrotic background is often a feature of high-grade carcinomas (**c**). Papanicolaou. Intermediate power.

Background

The background may reveal some important aspects of the lesion, such as a watery content in some cystic or papillary lesions, abundant mucus in mucocele-like lesions and mucinous carcinomas, or a coarse, granular proteinaceous material in lesions with a necrotic component (Fig. 7). In breast aspirates, the presence of necrosis is not a sign of stromal invasion, as it is a peculiar feature of high-grade ductal carcinoma in situ of the "comedo" type [see Chapter 8, this vol., pp. 68–93].

None of these morphological criteria alone is specific for either a benign or a malignant condition, but the presence of several consistent findings increases the diagnostic accuracy. Moreover, some authors suggest that the application of both cytological and architectural criteria is more reliable than cytology alone in distinguishing breast lesions [Dawson et al., 1995; Sneige and Staerkel, 1994].

Summary

General Cytological Features of Benign Lesions

- Large, single-layer sheets of uniform epithelial cells
- Small, round, homogeneous nuclei
- Even nuclear chromatin
- Small, single nucleoli
- Fair amount of cytoplasm
- Abundant myoepithelial cells and bipolar bare nuclei in the background

General Cytological Features of Malignant Lesions

- Small and irregular cell layers and 3-dimensional clusters
- Many intact single cells, loss of cohesion
- Different size and shape of the nuclei
- Irregular nuclear chromatin
- Prominent and/or multiple nucleoli
- Frequent and/or atypical mitotic figures

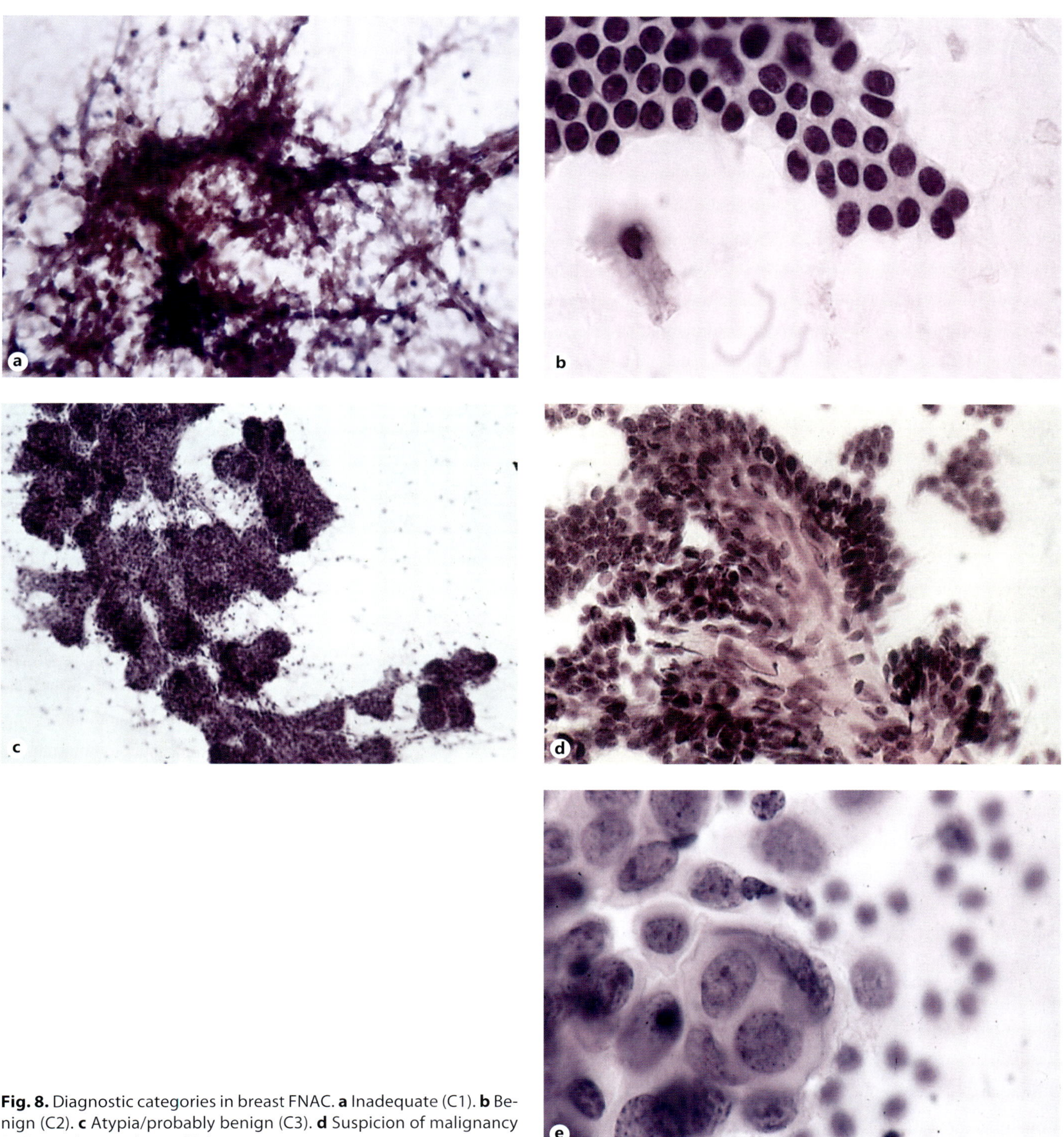

Fig. 8. Diagnostic categories in breast FNAC. **a** Inadequate (C1). **b** Benign (C2). **c** Atypia/probably benign (C3). **d** Suspicion of malignancy (C4). **e** Malignant lesion (C5).

Diagnostic Categories and Report

As early as 1996, the National Cancer Institute sponsored conference [1997] suggested the routine use of diagnostic categories in breast cytology. Similarly to the BI-RADS categories for radiological reporting, they summarize the results of the cytological diagnosis using a code, suggesting a management for that type of lesion. Different classifications exist, but most of them use a 5-tier coding system, which can virtually superimpose one classification on another (Fig. 8).

Classification
C1 Inadequate/Unsatisfactory
The sample is not contributory to the diagnosis, due to scant cellularity, air-drying artifacts, obscuring blood, inflammation, or other causes.

C2 Benign
A benign lesion can be safely diagnosed, or there is just no evidence of malignancy.

C3 Atypical/Indeterminate
The cytological findings are not diagnostic for the presence of high cellularity, equivocal cellular atypia, or aspects suggesting the presence of a borderline lesion, and the definite nature cannot be assessed based on cytology alone; this diagnostic category usually indicates the need for a more detailed diagnosis via biopsy or follow-up.

C4 Suspicious/Probably Malignant
Findings are highly suspicious of malignancy, but a definite diagnosis still cannot be made; in such cases, a biopsy is recommended to clarify the doubts before surgery.

C5 Malignant
The sample is diagnostic of a malignant neoplasm (if possible, specify the type).

A gray zone exists also in breast cytology. In certain cases, the need to resort to the categories of atypia/suspicion of malignancy is not due to the inability of a cytopathologist to recognize a specific entity but rather to the inherent nature of several breast lesions, such as proliferative disease or low-grade ductal carcinoma, which show equivocal aspects on cytology. These must not be too numerous, accounting for less than 20% (preferably 15%) of all cytological diagnoses according to the Non-Operative Diagnosis Subgroup of the National Coordinating Group for Breast Screening Pathology [2000].

In addition, inadequate cytology should not exceed 25% (preferably 15%); otherwise, another first-choice diagnostic technique, such as core needle biopsy, should be preferred. The specific requirements for adequacy have still not been defined. An adequate specimen obtained by FNAC is one that leads to the resolution of the problem presented by the breast lesion. It is mainly determined by the cytopathologist's opinion concerning the consistency between cytological and clinical/radiological findings and the quality of the cells present in the smear.

The use of a structured report improves the quality, clarity, and reproducibility of reports across departments, cities, and internationally. Moreover, it facilitates the communication between cytopathologists and clinicians, providing a helpful tool in patient management [Ellis and Srigley, 2016].

However, the cytology report must not be reduced to a code or diagnostic category and should include all the relevant information that allows to fully understand the diagnosis in a way similar to a surgical specimen or biopsy report [Field et al., 2016].

The cytology report should include at least:

- Description of smear cellularity (few, moderate, or abundant), which is a measure of the adequacy of the sample;
- Cytological description with all the relevant features and diagnostic criteria
- Statement of whether the lesion is completely benign (such as "no malignant cells are seen")
- Conclusion, containing a specific diagnosis or weighted differential diagnosis
- Code or diagnostic category

In the following chapters, the main cytological features of the different breast lesions will be discussed, as well as the most appropriate diagnostic category and management for specific diagnoses.

References

ACR BI-RADSs – Ultrasound; in: ACR Breast Imaging Reporting and Data System, Breast Imaging Atlas. Reston, American College of Radiology, 2003.

Ahmed I, Nazir R, Chaudhary MY, Kundi S: Triple assessment of breast lump. J Coll Physicians Surg Pak 2007;17:535–538.

Candelaria RP, Hwang L, Bouchard RR, Whitman GJ: Breast ultrasound: current concepts. Semin Ultrasound CT MR 2013;34:213–225.

D'Orsi CJ, Sickles EA, Mendelson EB, Morris EA, et al: ACR BI-RADS® Atlas, Breast Imaging Reporting and Data System. Reston, American College of Radiology 2013.

Dawson AE, Mulford DK, Sheils LA: The cytopathology of proliferative breast disease: comparison with features of ductal carcinoma in situ. Am J Clin Pathol 1995;103:438–442.

Ellis DW, Srigley J: Does standardised structured reporting contribute to quality in diagnostic pathology? The importance of evidence-based data sets. Virchows Arch 2016;468:51–59.

Field AS, Schmitt F, Vielh P: IAC standardized reporting of breast fine-needle aspiration biopsy cytology. Acta Cytol 2017;61:3–6.

Garud HT, Sheet D, Mahadevappa M, Chatterjee J, Kumar Ray A, Ghosh A: Breast fine needle aspiration cytology practices and commonly perceived diagnostic significance of cytological features: a pan-India survey. J Cytol 2012;29:183–189.

Irwig L, Macaskill P: Evidence relevant to guidelines for the investigation of breast symptoms. Woolloomooloo, National Breast Cancer Centre, 1997.

Kashyap A, Jain M, Shukla S, Andley M: Study of nuclear morphometry on cytology specimens of benign and malignant breast lesions: a study of 122 cases. J Cytol 2017;34:10–15.

Kline TS, Kline IK, Howell LP: Guides to Clinical Aspiration Biopsy. Breast. Philadelphia, Lippincott Williams & Wilkins, 1999.

Lim JC, Al-Masri H, Salhadar A, Xie HB, Gabram S, Wojcik EM: The significance of the diagnosis of atypia in breast FNA. Diagn Cytopathol 2004;31: 285–288.

National Cancer Institute sponsored conference: The uniform approach to breast fine-needle aspiration biopsy. Diagn Cytopathol 1997;16:295–311.

Non-Operative Diagnosis Subgroup of the National Coordinating Group for Breast Screening Pathology: Guidelines for Non-Operative Diagnostic Procedures and Reporting in Breast Cancer Screening. Sheffield, NHS Cancer Screening Programmes, 2001, NHSBSP Publ 50.

Sanders MA, Roland L, Sahoo S: Clinical implications of subcategorizing BI-RADS 4 breast lesions associated with microcalcification: a radiology-pathology correlation study. Breast J 2010;16:28–31.

Sneige N, Staerkel GA: Fine needle aspiration cytology of ductal hyperplasia with and without atypia and ductal carcinoma in situ. Hum Pathol 1994;25: 485–492.

Pinamonti M, Zanconati F: Breast Cytopathology. Assessing the Value of FNAC in the Diagnosis of Breast Lesions.
Monogr Clin Cytol. Basel, Karger, 2018, vol 24, pp 20–24 (DOI: 10.1159/000479764)

Normal Breast

Hints of Breast Anatomy and Histology

The mammary gland is located before the pectoral muscle and covered by skin. Normally, there are two mammary glands, one on either side of the sternum, but breast tissue or nipples may occur anywhere along the embryonic milk lines. The breast consists for the most part of adipose and connective tissue, enclosing a smaller proportion of glands. The glandular tissue consists of the lactiferous ducts and the so-called terminal ductal-lobular units (TDLUs), which are the morphological and functional unit of the breast gland. TDLUs comprise a lobule, which is a cluster of 10–100 sac-like acini with secretory function, and a terminal duct connecting it to the duct system (Fig. 1). TDLUs are surrounded by a loose connective tissue, sensitive to hormonal stimulation, and devoid of elastic fibers. This system of ducts, surrounded by dense connective tissue provided with elastic fibers, is composed of a series of ducts of increasing caliber. The latter converge towards the major lactiferous ducts, each of which drains a single breast segment. Each of the lactiferous ducts, in total a dozen, presents in its distal end a dilatation, called lactiferous sinus, before giving origin to a collecting duct, which opens with its own orifice in the nipple.

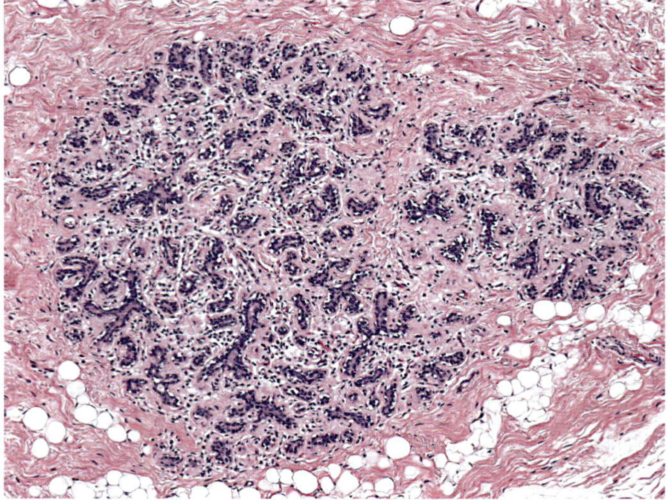

Fig. 1. Normal breast lobule. The terminal ductal-lobular unit is composed of 10–100 small acini connected to a terminal duct, which collects the mammary secretion into the milk duct system. The acini are enveloped by the intralobular stroma, a loose connective tissue sensitive to hormonal stimulation. H&E. Low power.

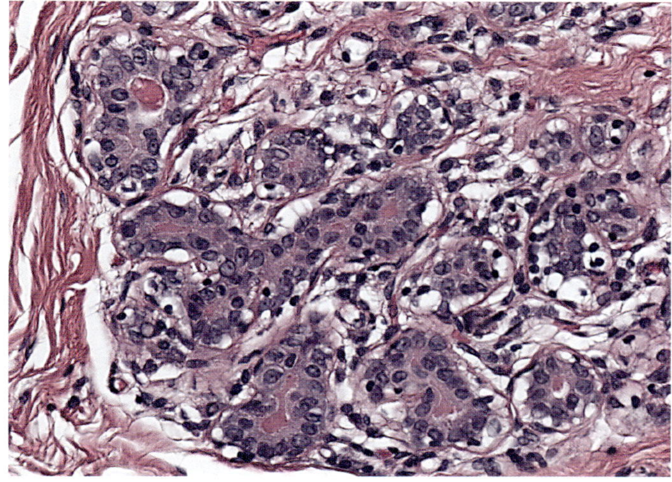

Fig. 2. Histology of normal ductal cells. Acini and ducts are coated internally by a double cellular layer. The inner layer is made up of cuboidal or cylindrical epithelial glandular cells, the ductal cells, while the outer layer is composed of myoepithelial cells. These cells have a small pyknotic nucleus and delicate cytoplasm which appears "empty" in histological preparations. H&E. High power.

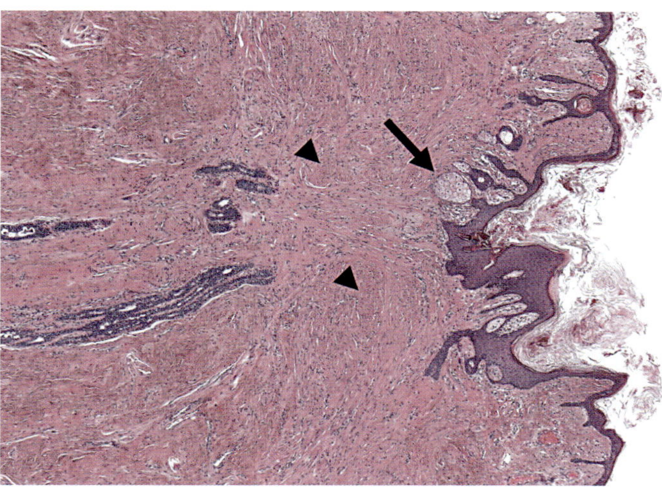

Fig. 3. Histology of the nipple. Breast secretion is collected through milk ducts into the nipple, where ductal epithelium is substituted by keratinized squamous epithelium. Here, sebaceous glands are present (arrow), and smooth muscle fibers are evident in the stroma (arrowheads). H&E. Scanning magnification.

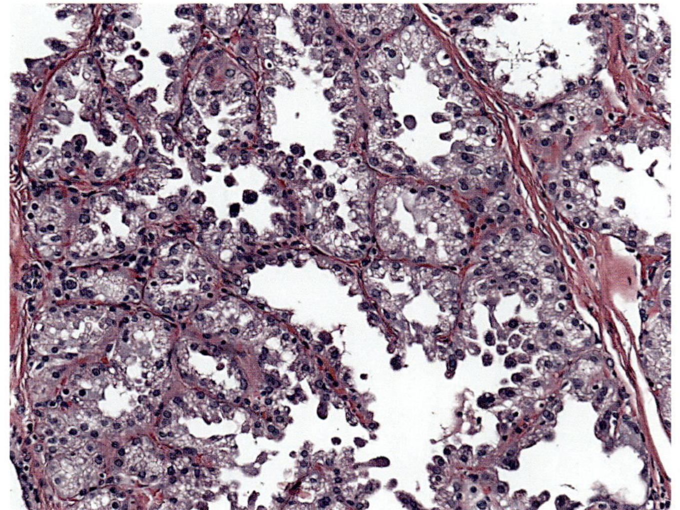

Fig. 4. Lactation changes in breast lobules. During late pregnancy and lactation, hormonal stimulation of breast tissue leads to an increase in size of the lobuli due to proliferation and functional activation of ductal cells. These cells increase in size and the cytoplasm becomes vacuolated; their active secretion results in the widening of acinar lumina, which are normally narrow and not easily seen (compare this picture with Fig. 2). H&E. Intermediate power.

A double layer of cells forms the epithelium of the mammary gland. The inner layer is composed of cylindrical or cubic glandular cells, named ductal cells, while the outer layer is composed of cells with the histochemical, immunohistochemical, and ultrastructural characteristics of myoepithelial cells (Fig. 2). In the nipple, where apocrine and sebaceous glands are also observed, the glandular epithelium is transformed into keratinized squamous epithelium (Fig. 3). Here, the fibrous stroma surrounding the ducts merges within the dermis and contains also the fibers of the erector muscle of the nipple.

Before puberty, the glandular breast tissue consists of a ductal system without TDLUs. In males, this aspect remains unchanged to adulthood, while it is subject to substantial changes in the female sex. During puberty, TDLUs develop and are already able to assume a secretory function. During pregnancy and lactation, the modifications include the increased number of TDLUs and secretory activity of the cells lining the lobules (Fig. 4). A secretory aspect can be observed, even if in less accentuated form, during the menstrual cycle. After menopause, TDLUs gradually disappear, and the mammary gland of an elderly woman comes down to fat tissue, connective tissue, and some residual lobules (Fig. 5).

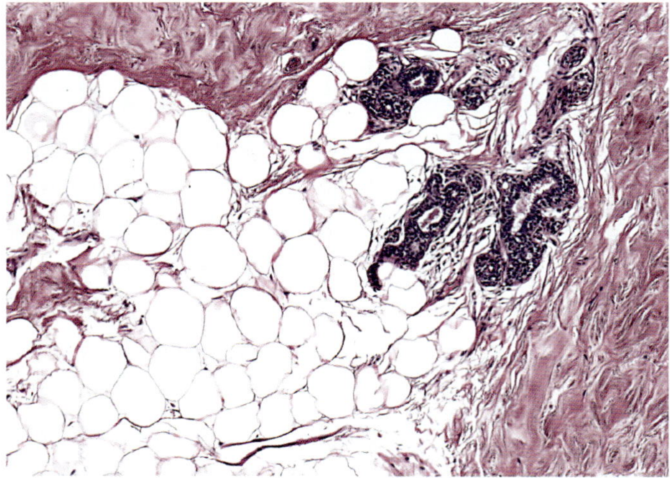

Fig. 5. Menopausal involution of the breast. In menopause, due to decreasing estrogenic stimulation, breast parenchyma progressively involutes, being gradually substituted by adipose tissue. Glandular tissue is represented by variably atrophic ducts and few residual acini, typically much smaller than those of a fertile woman (cf. Fig. 1). H&E. Low power.

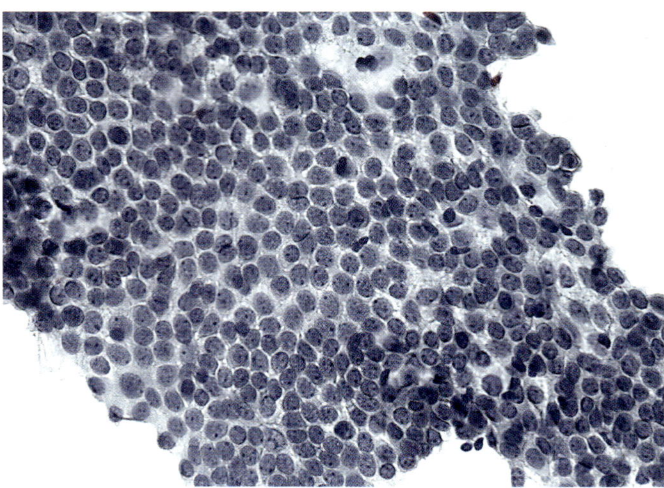

Fig. 6. Normal ductal cells. In cytological samples, ductal cells are usually arranged in cohesive single-layer sheets. They show uniform round nuclei with even chromatin distribution and often a single, small nucleolus. A thin rim of pale cytoplasm surrounds each nucleus, producing a regular "honeycomb" texture. Papanicolaou. High power.

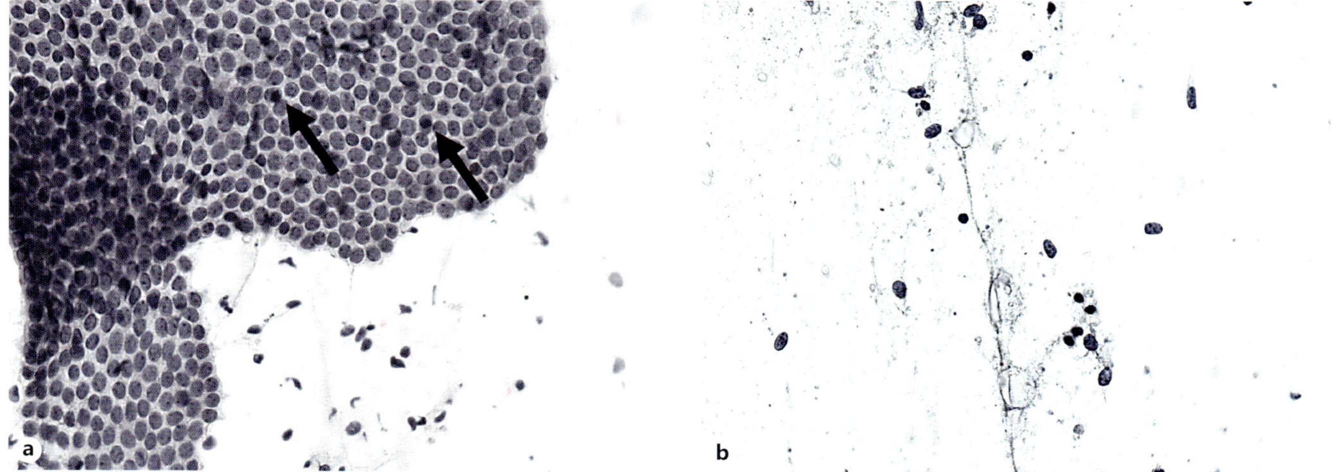

Fig. 7. Myoepithelial cells. Myoepithelial cells are visible above the ductal epithelial cells as scattered pyknotic dark nuclei (arrows) (**a**). Single bare oval (also called "bipolar") nuclei are visible in the background (**b**). They are considered an important sign of a benign condition. Papanicolaou. High power.

Cytology of the Normal Breast

The different cells forming each component of breast tissue might be found in a cytological smear due to the presence of normal breast tissue inside a lesion or an error in sampling. Remember that the presence of normal cells in the aspirate does not exclude malignancy, and all the cells in the smear have to be carefully examined, along with clinical and radiological information, before establishing the diagnosis.

Ductal cells should represent the vast majority of cells found in an aspirate from a benign epithelial lesion. They derive from the epithelial lining of breast ducts as well as

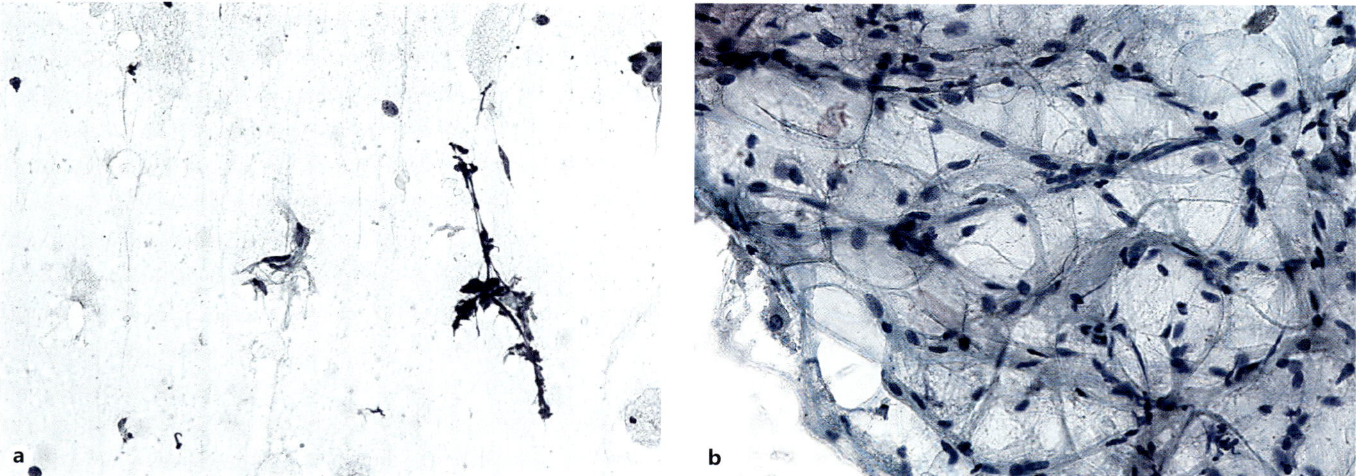

Fig. 8. Stromal cells. Scattered fibroblasts with elongated nuclei and spindle-shaped cell contours may be present in the background of a breast aspirate (**a**), but they are more commonly seen as components of stromal fragments alongside with adipocytes (**b**). Papanicolaou. High power.

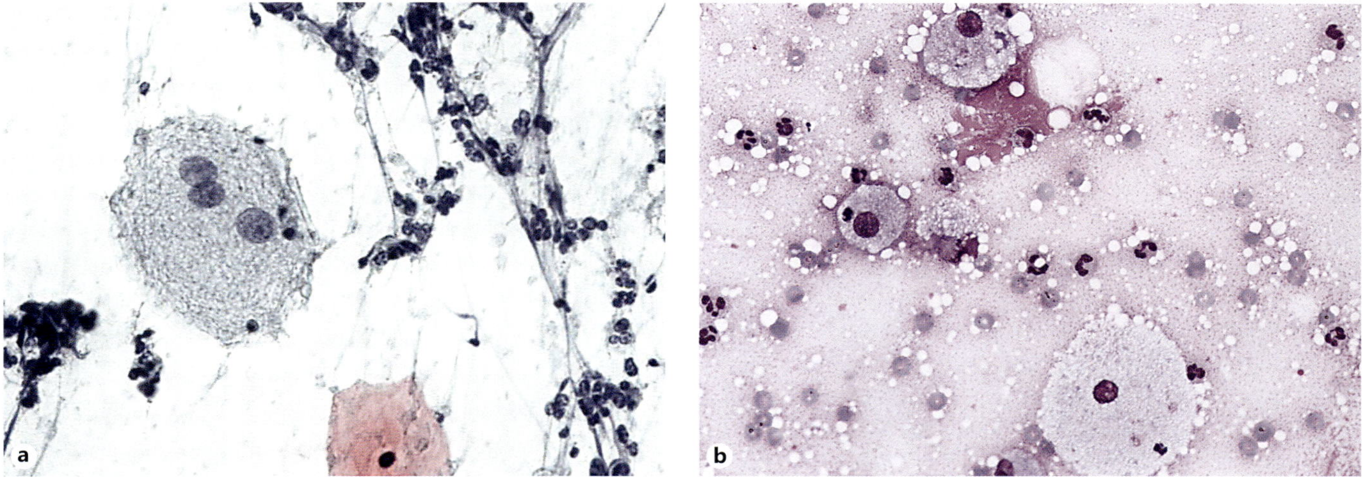

Fig. 9. Histiocytes. Histiocytes and macrophages are a common finding in breast lesions, especially in those with a cystic component or an ongoing reparative process (scars/steatonecrosis). Nuclei are round, oval, or beam shaped and have fine and homogeneous chromatin. The cytoplasm is wide and frequently contains cellular debris or multiple small vacuoles ("foamy" macrophages). Papanicolaou (**a**) and May-Grünwald-Giemsa (**b**). High power.

from TDLUs; they are relatively small, with round-shaped and uniform nuclei measuring approximately 8–10 μm in May-Grünwald-Giemsa or 7–8 μm in Papanicolaou staining. Nuclei have pale homogeneous chromatin and often a single, small nucleolus is visible. Cytoplasm is well appreciable in cellular layers, being absent or extremely scant in the occasional single cells (Fig. 6).

Cytologically, myoepithelial cells are visible as sparse small, dark, pyknotic nuclei above ductal cells in epithelial cell layers (Fig. 7). It is possible to visualize them by making small alternative changes in the microscope focus while looking at epithelial cell layers. Their presence is an important sign of a benign lesion, since it witnesses the intraepithelial nature of a proliferative process.

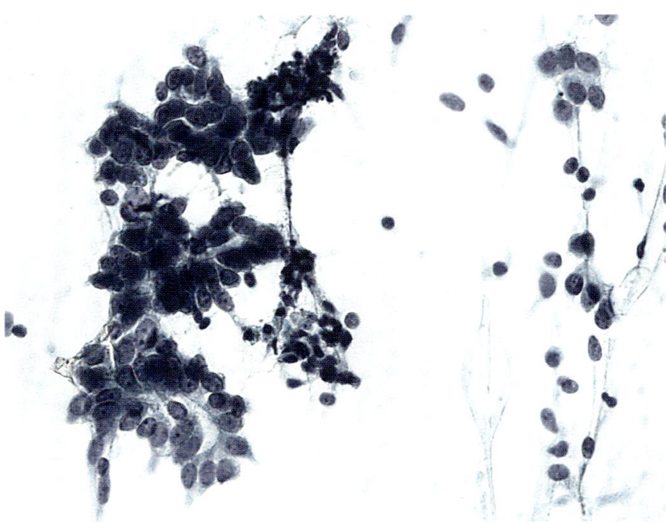

Fig. 10. Cytology of lactation changes. During pregnancy and lactation, the active ductal cells are enlarged and tend to lose their cohesiveness in the smear. Nuclei frequently show evident nucleoli, but the chromatin is fine and evenly distributed and nuclear contours are smooth. Papanicolaou. High power.

Bare or naked nuclei are often present next to epithelial cell layers. They are round or oval shaped (frequently referred as "bipolar" bare nuclei) and almost of the same size as ductal cells (Fig. 7). Whether they represent myoepithelial, stromal, or epithelial cells is somewhat controversial [Kline and Kline, 1989; Tsuchiya et al., 1987; Zajicek, 1971]. Most investigators have assumed that they are myoepithelial in origin, but a more recent study [Dabbs and Gown, 1999] has shown strong immunohistochemical support for a stromal origin of these cells. They are present in large quantity in fibroadenomas and are generally considered as a sign of a benign lesion.

Stromal cells are variably present in breast aspirates being difficult to extract from the tissue. They show thin, elongated nuclei and spindle-shaped, pale cytoplasm. They can present singly or are arranged in clusters with a relative quantity of amorphous proteinaceous material and without the typical honeycomb, ordered disposition of epithelial cells (Fig. 8).

Adipocytes may be present in breast aspirates, especially when FNAC is performed on adipose nodules or scar-like lesions and in adipose breasts. They have voluminous, transparent cytoplasm with well-demarcated contours and a small, peripherally located nucleus. They usually present in aggregates and assume a polyhedral shape due to reciprocal compression. They are better observed using May-Grünwald-Giemsa-stained preparations, since the alcoholic fixative causes the dissolution of adipose material.

Histiocytes and macrophages are typically present in aspirates from scar-like lesions, cysts, and duct ectasia, since they tend to accumulate in the dilated duct lumina. They show wide pale and often vacuolated cytoplasm and oval or bean-shaped nuclei with uniform chromatin. The cytoplasm may contain granules and cellular debris depending on the context in which they are found (Fig. 9).

Pregnancy- and lactation-related alterations in breast aspirates include nuclear enlargement, presence of evident nucleoli, and sometimes cytoplasmic vacuoles in ductal cells. Those cells tend to dissociate from epithelial cell layers and lose their cytoplasm, resulting in a greater amount of bare nuclei, which are more often round rather than bipolar and may contain large nucleoli (Fig. 10) [Finley et al., 1989].

References

Dabbs DJ, Gown AM: The distribution of calponin and smooth muscle myosin heavy chain in fine needle aspiration biopsies of the breast. Diagn Cytopathol 1999;20:203–207.

Finley JL, Silverman JF, Lannin DR: Fine-needle aspiration cytology of breast masses in pregnant and lactating women. Diagn Cytopathol 1989;5:255–259.

Kline TS, Kline IK: Other benign lesions; in Guides to Clinical Aspiration Biopsy: Breast. New York, Igaku-Shonin, 1989, pp 41–83.

Tsuchiya S, Maruyama Y, Koike Y, Yamada K, Kobayashi Y, Kagaya A: Cytologic characteristics and origin of naked nuclei in breast aspirate smears. Acta Cytol 1987;31:285–290.

Zajicek J: 7. Breast; in Zajicek J: Aspiration Biopsy Cytology. Part I: Cytology of Supradiaphragmatic Organs. Monogr Clin Cytol. Basel, Karger, 1974, vol 4, pp 136–194.

Pinamonti M, Zanconati F: Breast Cytopathology. Assessing the Value of FNAC in the Diagnosis of Breast Lesions.
Monogr Clin Cytol. Basel, Karger, 2018, vol 24, pp 25–32 (DOI: 10.1159/000479765)

Cytology of Inflammatory and Reactive Changes

Many inflammatory and reactive breast lesions may clinically and radiologically mimic cancer and be subjected to FNAC to exclude malignancy. Aspirates from lesions discussed in this chapter are variably characterized by the presence of inflammatory cells, which include granulocytes, lymphocytes, histiocytes, and multinucleated giant cells. The cytopathologist has the task of identifying the most probable nature (and if possible the cause) of the inflammatory process and of carefully looking for atypical cells in order to exclude with sufficient accuracy a concomitant neoplasm, since breast cancer and infection may coexist [Demay, 1996]. The inflammatory process might alter epithelial cells present on the smear, which may show evident nucleoli and nuclear enlargement, thus aspirates from this kind of lesions frequently fall into the "atypical" (C3) or "suspicious" (C4) diagnostic category.

In investigating inflammatory lesions, cytology may benefit from the combination with microbiologic cultural examination. The presence of a negative culture does not exclude infection, but a positive culture can direct the therapy and result in true benefits for the patients.

Acute Inflammation/Breast Abscesses

Acute mastitis is uncommon and typically presents during lactation due to ulcerations of the areolar skin and subsequent infection by the bacteria of the skin flora (mainly *Staphylococcus* and *Streptococcus* spp.). Abscess formation can lead to the appearance of a mass in the breast, which is typically painful and surmounted by red skin. Mammography is rarely done in this situation due to the lactating status of the patient and the pain provoked by the device. Ultrasound is not specific, showing an ill-defined hypoechoic mass, and the diagnosis is usually made through an "ex iuvantibus" policy.

FNAC is sometimes performed on breast abscesses in patients in whom first-line antibiotic treatment does not work properly or when a residual mass is found after the resolution of the symptoms. The aspirated material is typically purulent, and many neutrophils are evident in the smear, associated to a variable number of histiocytes, scant lymphocytes, and occasional epithelial cells altered by the inflammatory process (Fig. 1) [Das et al., 1992]. Reactive squamous metaplastic cells might be present as well.

Chronic Inflammation

When acute mastitis does not resolve, it might evolve into chronic inflammation. This eventuality is often associated with fibrosis and the architectural remodeling that results in duct ectasia [see Chapter 5, this vol., pp. 33–40]. The chronic infiltrate is made up of lymphocytes, plasma cells, and some residual neutrophils. The fibrotic reaction accompanying the process may mimic cancer on both clinical exam-

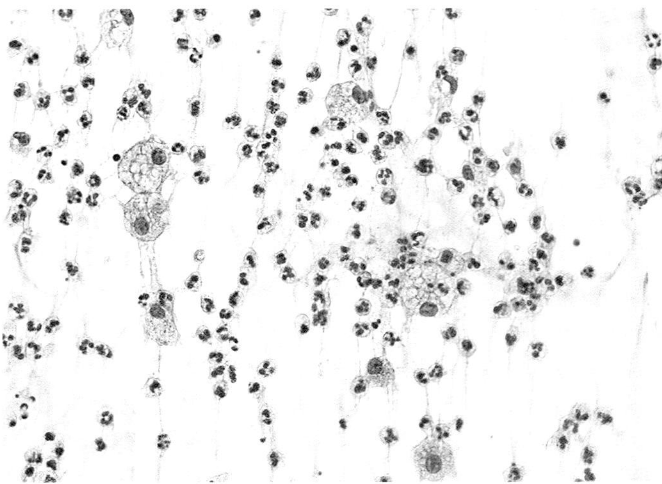

Fig. 1. Acute mastitis. This aspirate was taken from a sonographically suspicious lesion behind the nipple of a lactating woman. Numerous dispersed neutrophil granulocytes are visible admixed with some foamy macrophages in a "watery" background. Diagnostic category: C2 (benign). Papanicolaou. High power.

ination and mammogram/ultrasound and may result in a paucicellular or inadequate aspirate. In such cases, core needle biopsy is recommended, especially if rare atypical cells are detected on the smear.

Granulomatous Reactions

The presence of multinucleated giant cells in an aspirate indicates the presence of a granulomatous reaction. Breast granulomas may result from many different conditions, including tuberculosis, sarcoidosis, fungal infections, cat scratch disease, foreign body reactions, subareolar abscesses, duct ectasia, and idiopathic causes [Das et al., 1992].

Microbiological cultures are extremely useful when dealing with granulomatous breast lesions, since they allow diagnosing tuberculosis among a large number of other entities sharing similar aspects on cytological smears. Anyway, we stress the importance of an accurate clinical investigation, which can explain the presence of a granulomatous reaction in most cases without the need of other ancillary techniques.

Foreign Body Reactions

Foreign bodies are the most common cause of breast granulomas. Women with silicone breast implants, whether aesthetic or due to a previous mastectomy with prosthetic reconstruction, may develop periprosthetic granulomas due to microscopic rupture of the implants and the leak of silicone in the adjacent tissue. This occurrence is relatively frequent and is correlated to the aging of the implant [Brown et al., 1997]. Silicone granulomas (also called "siliconomas") usually appear on ultrasound as nodular hyperechoic masses with fine internal echoes, but they might be hypoechoic and simulate other lesions, such as fibroadenomas or cancer. This eventuality must be carefully excluded, especially in patients previously treated with mastectomy that are at high risk of developing local recurrences. FNAC performed on siliconomas typically shows giant multinucleated cells with cytoplasmic vacuoles containing birefringent particles (Fig. 2). Silicone may migrate to other sites, and the same cells might be present in aspirates from axillary lymph nodes. Silicone adenopathy in the absence of evident local rupture has also been reported [Brown et al., 1997].

Other foreign bodies capable of generating granulomatous reactions in the breast include suture fibers from previous surgery and carbon injected in the site of a lesion to be excised. Identifying microscopic particles of the foreign body in the cytoplasm of giant cells allows the cytopathologist to make a definitive diagnosis (Fig. 2).

Tuberculosis

Primitive breast tuberculosis is an extremely rare entity in western countries, comprising 0.1% of all tuberculosis cases [Thompson et al., 1997]. Nevertheless, it is more common in developing countries, where tuberculosis is endemic, and its occurrence might increase significantly due to immigration from those countries. It simulates breast cancer clinically, with firm masses that may cause skin retraction and eventually ulceration, and symptoms of systemic tuberculosis might be absent. Aspirates show large multinucleated giant cells that typically display numerous nuclei arranged in a circle or horseshoe at the periphery of the cytoplasm (Langerhans cells) admixed with lymphocytes and neutrophils in a necrotic background [Tse et al., 2003]. Staining for acid-fast bacilli or Ziehl-Neelsen staining may be useful to highlight the presence of mycobacteria in the smear [Mistry et al., 2012].

Sarcoidosis

Sarcoidosis is an idiopathic systemic granulomatous disease that may rarely present as palpable mass in the breast simulating invasive cancer [Gisvold et al., 2000]. The contemporary presence of nodular masses in axillary lymph

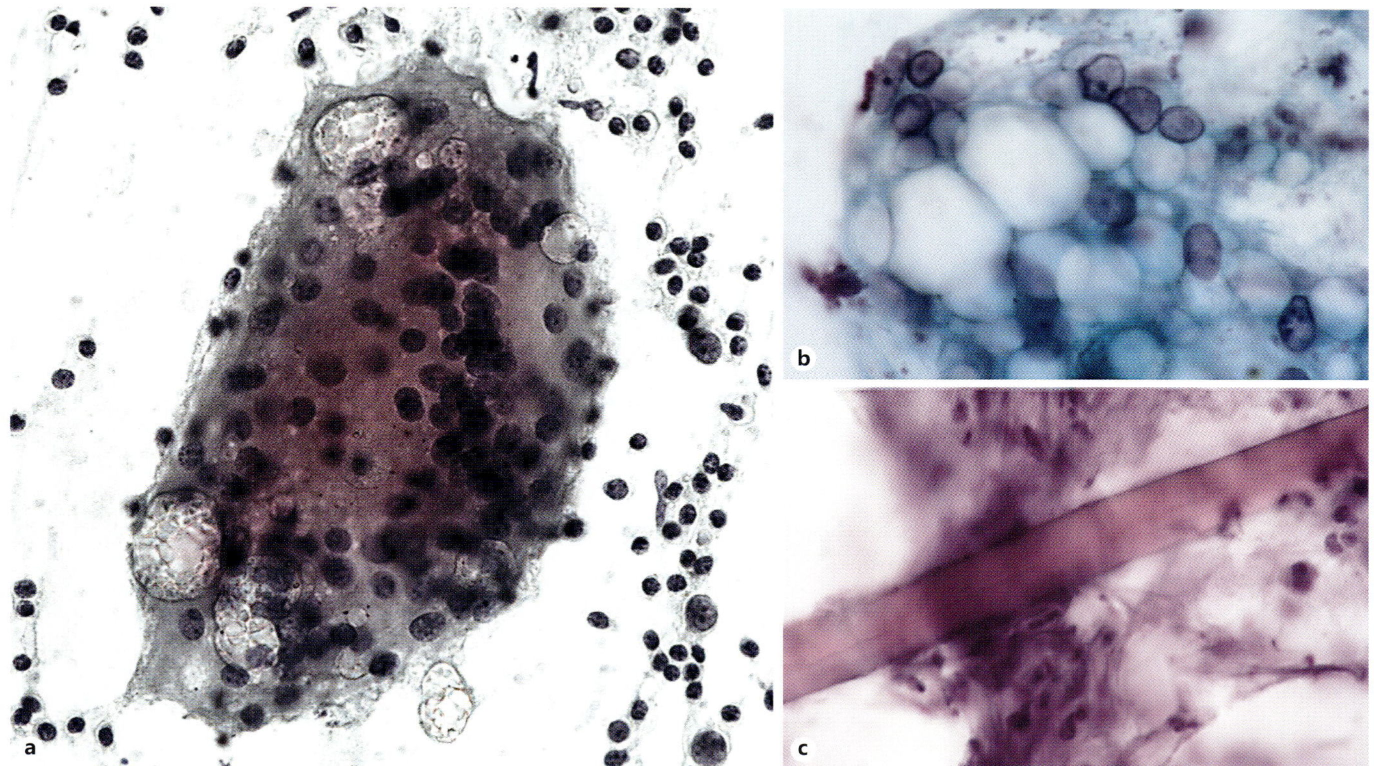

Fig. 2. Foreign body reactions. A large multinucleated giant cell with silicone particles in the cytoplasm (**a**); multinucleated giant cells intervene also in the reparation process after breast surgery, trying to phagocyte adipose tissue (**b**) and suture fibers (**c**). Papanicolaou. High power.

nodes and lungs might be very suggestive of a metastatic breast carcinoma, so FNAC or core needle biopsy can play a fundamental role in the diagnosis and management of such cases [Zujić et al., 2015]. Aspirates from sarcoidosis granulomas display multinucleated giant cells of the Langerhans type, but unlike tuberculosis, the background is clear and lacks caseating necrosis. *Asteroid bodies* in the cytoplasm of these cells are a curious finding that have been described in association with sarcoidosis but are not exclusive of this condition.

Idiopathic Lobular Granulomatous Mastitis

Idiopathic lobular granulomatous mastitis is another rare cause of granulomas in the breast. It may occur in women between 20 and 40 years of age, typically in the aftermath of a pregnancy, and it is bilateral in 25% of cases. Granulomas are located in breast lobules and coexist with multiple microabscesses. Aspirates typically display epithelioid histiocytes admixed with fibroblasts and neutrophils in a nonnecrotic background and may lack multinucleated giant cells. This is a diagnosis of exclusion and should be taken into consideration when all other known causes of granulomatous inflammation have been excluded [Tse et al., 2003].

Steatonecrosis

Steatonecrosis or fat necrosis is a possible complication following trauma, surgery, or radiotherapy in the breast. It is more frequent in overweight women and typically presents as a painless, firm, and relatively circumscribed palpable mass, on average 2 cm in diameter, which may cause retraction or dimpling of the overlying skin and alter the subjective sensation of a preexistent scar. This aspect is quite suspicious, especially in patients already treated for breast cancer that are at high risk of local recurrence. Mammography shows a spiculated, poorly defined mass that may contain punctuate or large irregular calcifications [Hogge et al., 1995]. Ultrasound typically reveals a suspicious, irregular and inhomogeneous mass that may contain cystic spaces;

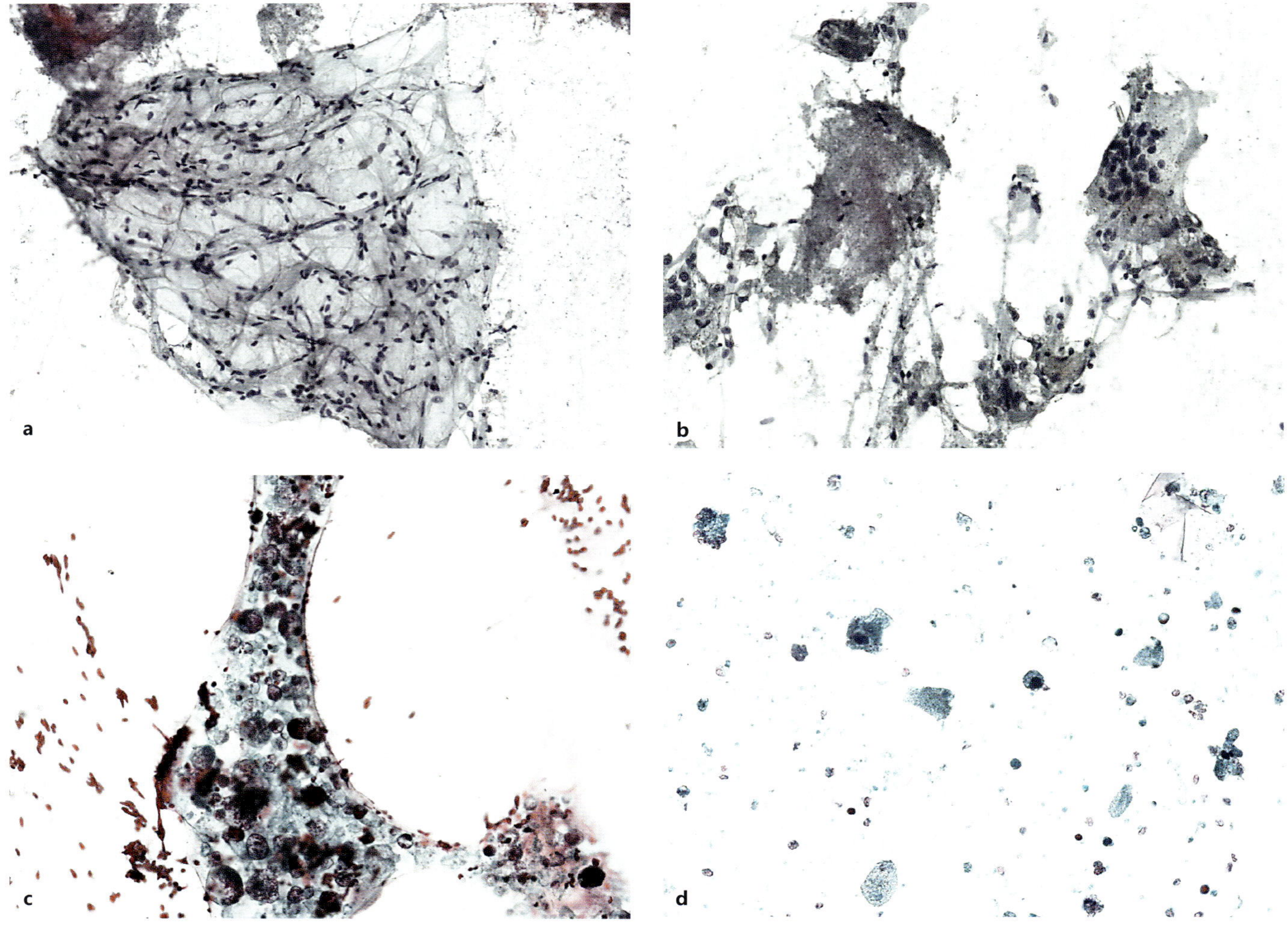

Fig. 3. Steatonecrosis. Aspirates from areas of steatonecrosis vary widely, but frequently display some peculiar features, including fibro-adipose stromal fragments (**a**), necrotic debris, and foreign-body giant cells (**b**). Hemosiderin-laden and foamy macrophages may indicate the presence of hemorrhagic areas and cystic spaces, respectively (**c**, **d**). Papanicolaou. **a–c** Intermediate power. **d** High power.

therefore, FNAC is frequently called upon to clearly define this worrisome lesion.

Aspirates from areas of steatonecrosis are typically loosely cellular, often showing a dirty granular background, fatty tissue fragments, and variable amounts of inflammatory cells. Foamy or hemosiderin-laden macrophages may result from the presence of cystic areas or previous hemorrhages. The disruption of adipose tissue and the presence of cholesterol crystals may generate a foreign-body granulomatous reaction, and thus multinucleated giant cells can also be present in the smear (Fig. 3, 4). Some free lipid droplets might be seen as empty spaces in the granular background, eventually surrounded by blood cells.

Epithelial cells might be present in an aspirate from an area of steatonecrosis, but they are usually limited to a few small clusters and do not exhibit significant atypia.

Histiocytes in the aspirate may simulate isolated cancer cells, especially when considered in such a dirty background, but the nuclear chromatin is evenly distributed, and the nuclei have an oval or bean-like shape without significant membrane irregularities. The cytoplasm is typically broad, pale, and ill defined, and contains many small vesicles, different from the single, sharply demarcated vacuole that may be found in cancer cells from a lobular or secretory carcinoma (Fig. 5).

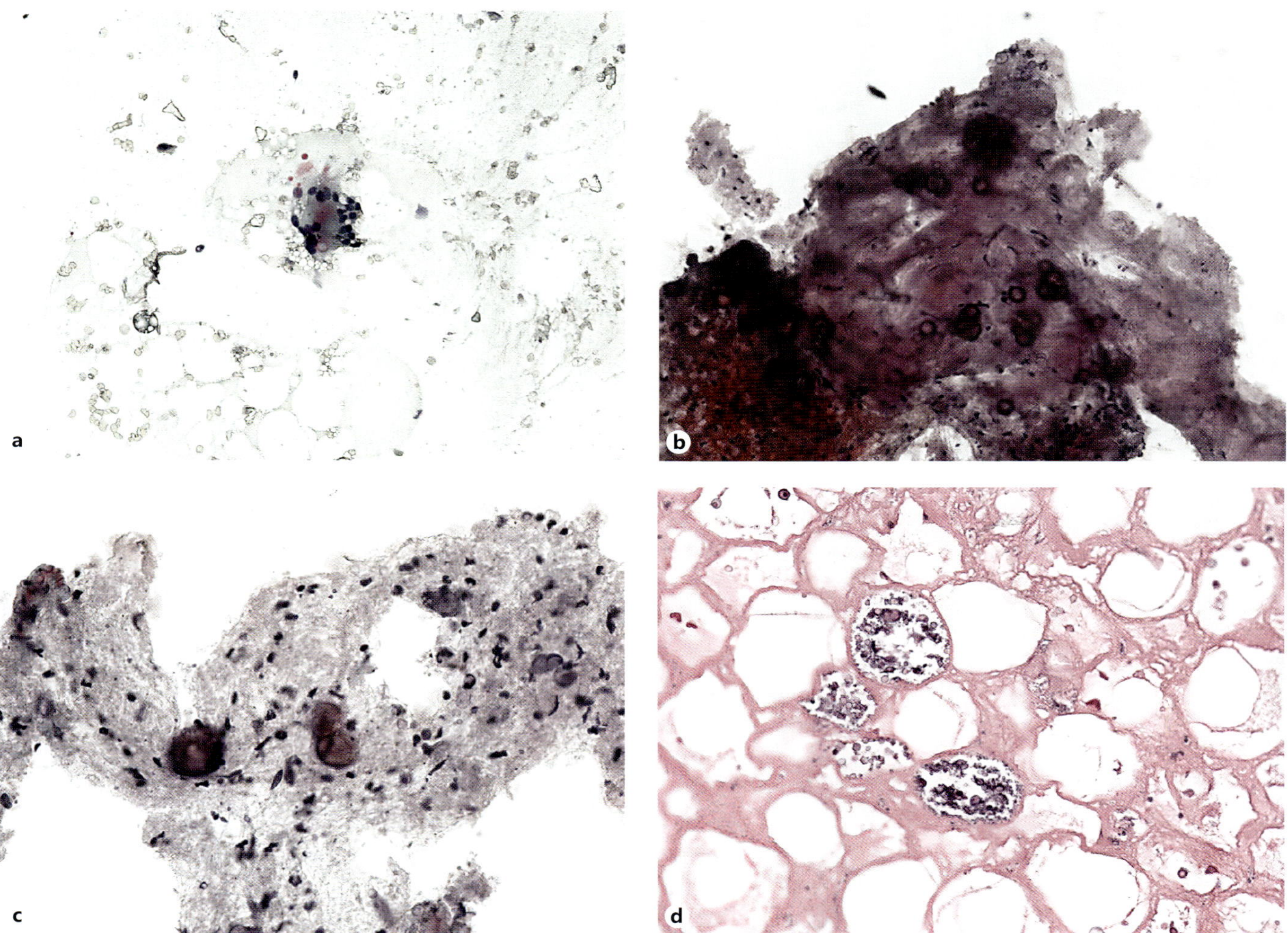

Fig. 4. Steatonecrosis. This case was taken from a patient who suffered blunt force trauma to the breast and developed a spiculated and ill-defined lesion which was considered suspicious through mammogram and ultrasound. The aspirate showed multinucleated giant cells and necrotic debris (**a**), including hemosiderin and some microcalcifications (**b**, **c**). The same peculiar features were also evident on histological evaluation of the resection specimen (**d**). Papanicolaou (**a–c**) and H&E (**d**). High power.

It is important to stress that fat necrosis and cancer can occur together. Therefore, the presence of aspects suggestive for steatonecrosis in the aspirate or in a biopsy specimen does not completely exclude the possibility of malignancy [Demay, 1996]. Fat necrosis is a dynamic process and should begin to resolve in a short time; thus, a brief period (<1 month) of watchful waiting after FNAC may resolve any question of malignancy [Nemenqani and Yaqoob, 2009].

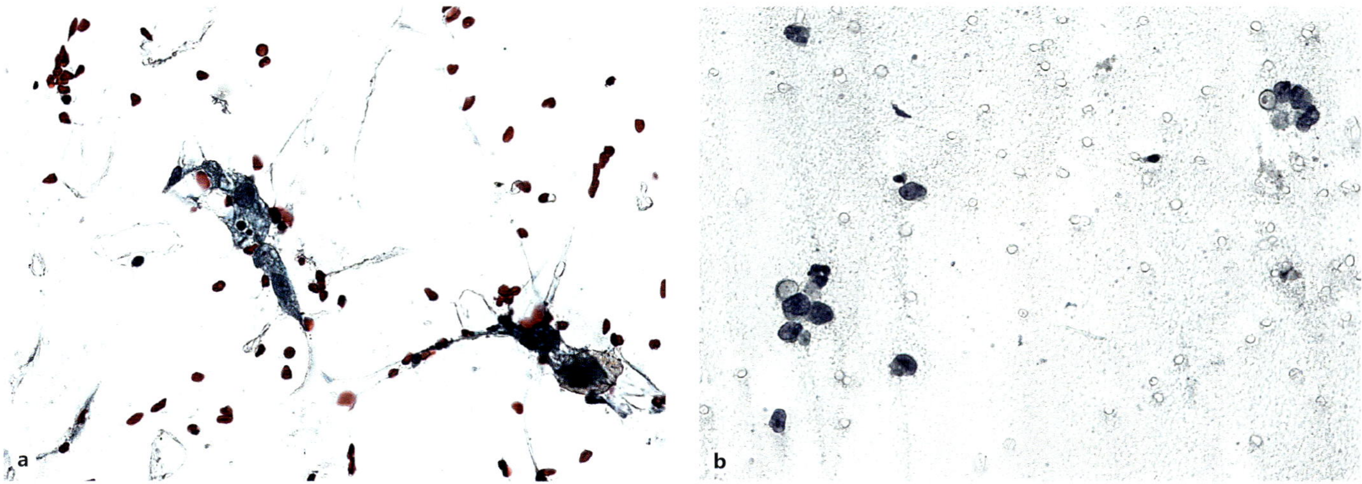

Fig. 5. Comparison between macrophages and cancer cells. Scattered macrophages present in areas of steatonecrosis might be mistaken as cancer cells, especially those of a lobular or secretory carcinoma, which have similar size and may show cytoplasmic vacuoles. Macrophages have round or oval-shaped nuclei with evenly distributed chromatin and inconspicuous nucleoli, and broad, pale, and ill-defined cytoplasm, which may contain multiple small vacuoles (**a**). Conversely, lobular carcinoma cells usually show nuclear atypia and have scanty cytoplasm with a single vacuole (**b**). Papanicolaou. High power.

Summary

Key Cytological Features of Steatonecrosis

- Scant cellularity
- Histiocytes, including foamy cells, siderophages, and multinucleated giant cells
- Variable number of other inflammatory cells
- Fragments of normal and/or degenerated adipose tissue
- Granular debris in the background

Common Pitfalls of FNA: Steatonecrosis

- Epithelioid macrophages in a necrotic background (cancer cells?)
- Many multinucleated giant cells (tuberculosis or other granulomatous diseases)
- Rare atypical cells masquerade as fat necrosis

Inflammatory Pseudotumor

This rare tumor-like entity is defined as a nodular lesion consisting of interlacing bundles of myofibroblastic cells with a prominent inflammatory infiltrate composed mainly of plasma cells and lymphocytes, which can mimic malignancy both clinically and radiologically [Zardawi et al., 2003]. Its precise etiology is unknown, being probably a reactive condition secondary to previous trauma or infection [Sari et al., 2011], and it may be considered as an exaggerated histiocytic reaction to fat necrosis in the breast [Sciallis et al., 2012].

Histologically, it appears as a distinct spindle cell proliferation of macrophages mimicking spindle cell neoplasms, such as sarcomatoid breast carcinoma and sarcomas. These cells have the immunohistochemical and ultrastructural characteristics of myofibroblasts [Gobbi et al., 1999]. Three major patterns have been described: myxoid/vascular, compact spindle cells, and hypocellular fibrous pattern, which can present in varying amounts in the same lesion [Hill, 2010; Sari et al., 2011].

FNAC shows loosely cohesive fragments of histiocytic cells with abundant, vacuolated cytoplasm, ill-defined cytoplasmic borders, and nuclei with small, prominent nucleoli, admixed with a variable amount of plasma cells, lymphocytes, and eosinophils (Fig. 6). Many spindle cells are present, isolated or as part of variably cellular stromal fragments. These cells may rarely look atypical and show mitoses, but they are not "pleomorphic" as in most high-grade sarcomas and spindle cell metaplastic carcinomas [Akbulut et al., 2007].

The highly suspicious radiologic and clinical aspects appear to be discordant with the relatively benign cytology; thus, most of these lesions undergo core needle biopsy and are then frequently excised, since none of these diagnostic

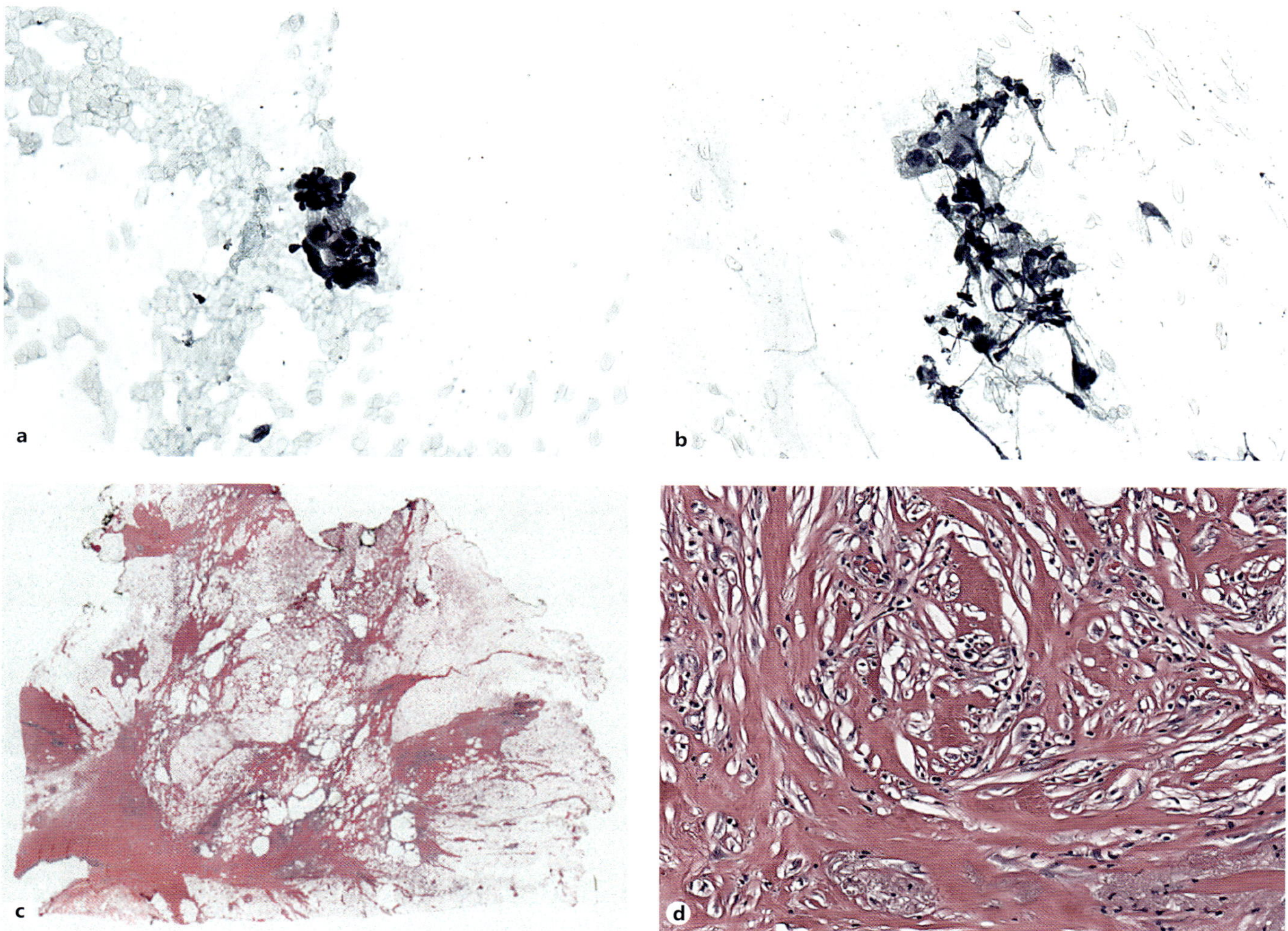

Fig. 6. Inflammatory pseudotumor. This case was taken from a 70-year-old patient previously treated with conservative surgery for intraductal carcinoma, who developed a suspicious mass at the site of surgery. The aspirate was loosely cellular, showing few aggregates composed of spindle-shaped histiocytic cells without cytological atypia clustered with some small lymphocytes (**a**, **b**). In the absence of epithelial cells and due to the impossibility of excluding a malignant neoplasm, which was strongly suspected by ultrasound, the aspirate was prudently assessed as unsatisfactory (C1) and the patient referred for further diagnostic examinations. Since a discordance still occurred after the benign results of the biopsy, the patient was treated with nodule resection. Histological evaluation showed proliferation of spindle cells without cytological atypia in a sclerotic stroma (**c**, **d**). The proliferation index was low, and the process was definitely considered reactive. Papanicolaou (**a**, **b**) and H&E (**c**, **d**). **a**, **b** High power. **c** Slide overview. **d** Intermediate power.

methods is capable of definitely excluding malignancy, and the whole lesion has to be carefully examined. Inflammatory pseudotumor is essentially a diagnosis of exclusion that can be made on the surgical specimen after all causes of granulomatous inflammation and spindle cell proliferation have been actively excluded. However, the diagnosis of inflammatory pseudotumor may be suspected when cytological examination reveals a hypercellular mostly bland spindle cell smear with a definitely histiocytic and sometimes plasmocytic component.

References

Akbulut M, Gunhan-Bilgen I, Zekioglu O, Duyqulu G, Oktay A, Ozdemir N: Fine needle aspiration cytology of inflammatory myofibroblastic tumour (inflammatory pseudotumour) of the breast: a case report and review of the literature. Cytopathology 2007;18:384–387.

Brown SL, Silverman BG, Berg WA: Rupture of silicone-gel breast implants: causes, sequelae, and diagnosis. Lancet 1997;350:1531–1537.

Das DK, Sodhani P, Kashyap V, Parkash S, Pant JN, Bhatnagar P: Inflammatory lesions of the breast: diagnosis by fine needle aspiration. Cytopathology 1992;3:281–289.

DeMay RM: Diseases and conditions of the breast; in Demay RM: The Art and Science of Cytopathology: Aspiration Cytology. Chicago, American Society of Clinical Pathologists, 1996, pp 856–859.

Gisvold JJ, Crotty TB, Johnson RE: Sarcoidosis presenting as spiculated breast masses. Mayo Clin Proc 2000;75:293–295.

Gobbi H, Atkinson JB, Kardos TF, Simpson JF, Page DL: Inflammatory myofibroblastic tumour of the breast: report of a case with giant vacuolated cells. Breast 1999;8:135–138.

Hill PA: Inflammatory pseudotumor of the breast: a mimic of breast carcinoma. Breast J 2010;16:549–550.

Hogge JP, Robinson RE, Magnant CM, et al: The mammographic spectrum of fat necrosis of the breast. Radiographics 1995;15:1347–1356.

Mistry Y, Ninama GL, Mistry K, Rajat R, Parmar R, Godhani A: Efficacy of fine-needle aspiration cytology, Ziehl-Neelsen stain and culture (BACTEC) in diagnosis of tuberculosis lymphadenitis. Nat J Med Res 2012;2:77–80.

Nemenqani D, Yaqoob N: Fine needle aspiration cytology of inflammatory breast lesions. J Pak Med Assoc 2009;59:167–170.

Sari A, Yigit S, Peker Y, Morgul Y, Coskun G, Cin N: Inflammatory pseudotumor of the breast. Breast J 2011;17:312–314.

Sciallis AP, Chen B, Folpe AL: Cellular spindled histiocytic pseudotumor complicating mammary fat necrosis: a potential diagnostic pitfall. Am J Surg Pathol 2012;36:1571–1578.

Thompson KS, Donzelli J, Jensen J, Pachucki C, Eng AM, Reyes CV: Breast and cutaneous mycobacteriosis: diagnosed by fine-needle aspiration biopsy. Diagn Cytopathol 1997;17:45–49.

Tse GM, Poon CS, Law BK, Pang LM, Chu WC, Ma TK: Fine needle aspiration cytology of granulomatous mastitis. J Clin Pathol 2003;56:519–521.

Zardawi IM, Clark D, Williamsz G: Inflammatory myofibroblastic tumor of the breast. A case report. Acta Cytol 2003;47:1077–1081.

Zujić PV, Grebić D, Valenčićc L: Chronic granulomatous inflammation of the breast as a first clinical manifestation of primary sarcoidosis. Breast Care (Basel) 2015;10:51–53.

Pinamonti M, Zanconati F: Breast Cytopathology. Assessing the Value of FNAC in the Diagnosis of Breast Lesions.
Monogr Clin Cytol. Basel, Karger, 2018, vol 24, pp 33–40 (DOI: 10.1159/000479766)

Cystic Lesions

Cystic lesions of the breast are an extremely common finding, especially in premenopausal women, and they are frequently symptomatic due to the presence of swelling and pain associated to the proliferative phase of the menstrual cycle, abnormal nipple discharge, or the occurrence of palpable lumps.

The common denominator of this group of lesions is the presence of fluid, amorphous material, and foamy histiocytes in the cytological smear without significant epithelial proliferation. Even if cystic lesions are almost always classified as benign, a cystic component might render an underlying cancer less evident.

Cysts are well studied with ultrasound, which shows anechoic lesions with regular margins, sharp anterior and posterior walls, and posterior enhancement (Fig. 1). The term "complex" cyst is used if there are echoes inside the cyst, reflecting the presence of a dense content or a papillary proliferation. FNAC is required to inspect all nonsimple cystic lesions and sometimes as a therapeutic means to empty symptomatic simple cysts.

Cysts

Introduction/Epidemiology

Cysts are the most common breast lesions, representing 10–15% of benign breast lesions. They can be found isolated or be part of fibrocystic changes (see below).

Cutaneous invagination of a collecting duct in the areolar region might result in an epidermoid cyst. These common lesions are prone to infectious events and be the site of acute inflammation, which may make the cyst adherent to the skin and appear clinically and sonographically suspicious.

Histological Features

Cysts are composed of a fibrous wall that may be lined by a cuboidal single-layer glandular epithelium or by apocrine metaplastic cells (apocrine cysts). The epithelial layer may be absent due to the internal pressure in the cyst. The content may consist of serous fluid or lipoproteinaceous dense material, sometimes comprising detached epithelial cells or foamy histiocytes (Fig. 2).

Cytology

The macroscopic aspect of the material aspired from a cyst is variable and can help in the final interpretation of the case. Simple cysts usually contain a clear, light yellow, or pink fluid, while a dense whitish and smelly material is usually indicative of an epidermal cyst. Sometimes the liquid may appear turbid, brown, green, or blue (blue-domed cysts) due to the presence of variably degenerated blood material.

Microscopically, the aspirate is characterized by amorphous, proteinaceous material and a variable amount of histiocytes with foamy cytoplasm (Fig. 3). An epithelial component may be absent or represented by layers of uniform ductal cells or apocrine metaplastic cell aggregates (Fig. 4).

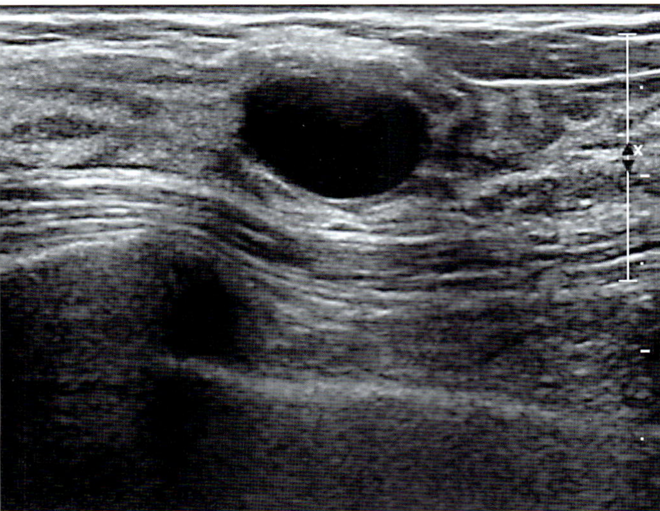

Fig. 1. Ultrasound imaging of a simple cyst. The lesion has liquid content and appears anechoic, with sharp contours and posterior enhancement.

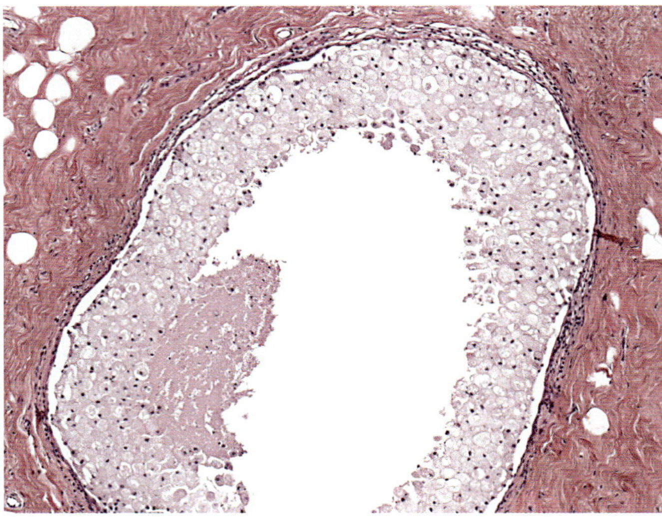

Fig. 2. Simple cyst. The wall of this small cyst is fibrous, and the epithelial layer is completely absent. Numerous foamy histiocytes are evident in the periphery of the lesion, while proteinaceous material is present in the center. H&E. Low power.

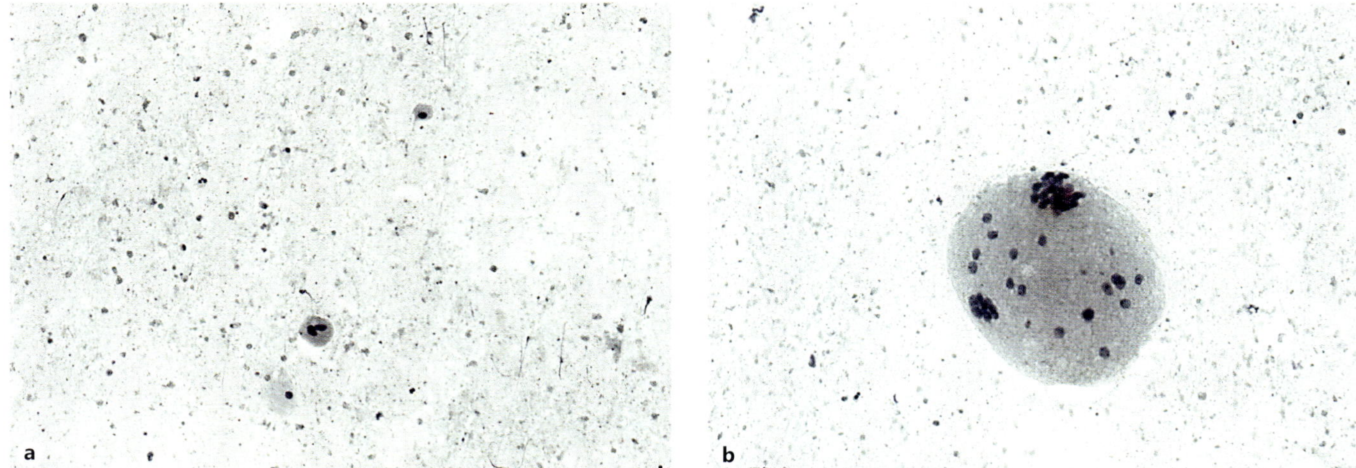

Fig. 3. Cytology of a simple cyst. Scattered histiocytes with foamy cytoplasm (**a**), sometimes multinucleated (**b**), are seen in a proteinaceous background. These multinucleated cells have their nuclei mainly clustered at one border of the cytoplasm and must be distinguished from the Langerhans-type giant cells of granulomatous processes. Papanicolaou. **a**, **b** Intermediate power.

Apocrine cells have round or oval-shaped nuclei with a small, single nucleolus and abundant granular cytoplasm in the presence of numerous mitochondria, which appear blue with Giemsa and reddish on Papanicolaou (Pap) stains (Fig. 5). They form variably sized layers or groups with a tendency to dissociation and typically lacking myoepithelial cells. Scant blood cells are frequently present, and hemosiderin can be seen as dark blue (May-Grünwald-Giemsa) or brown (Pap) granules in the cytoplasm of histiocytes (siderophages) revealing previous intracystic hemorrhages.

Aspirates from epidermal cysts display keratin anucleated squames, frequently admixed with inflammatory

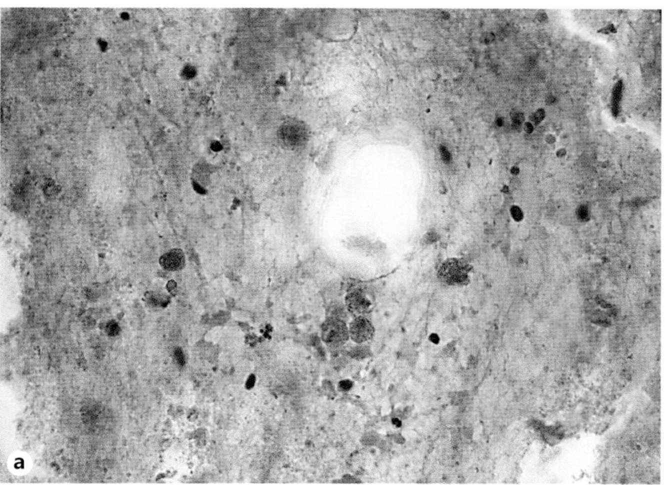

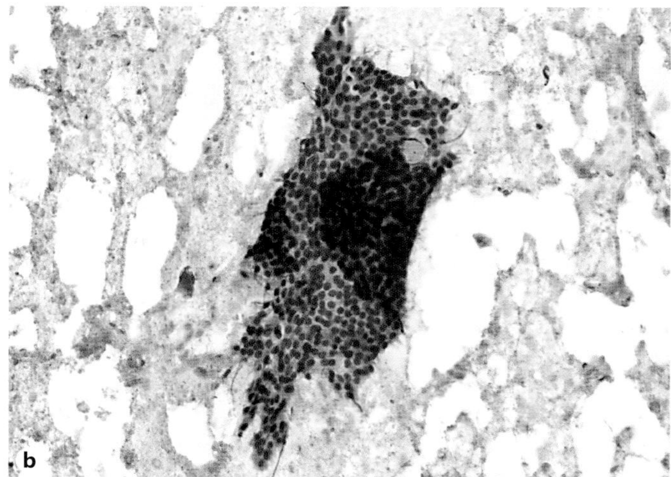

Fig. 4. Dense cyst. Some long-lasting cysts might have their content dehydrated and become denser. These cysts may be misinterpreted as solid lesions by ultrasound and undergo FNAC to exclude malignancy. Aspirates typically show a dense proteinaceous background and often some scattered macrophages (**a**) or benign epithelial cell layers (**b**), or may be completely acellular. Papanicolaou. Intermediate power.

cells, while immature keratinocytes are an uncommon finding. Keratin squames may appear bluish, carmine, or transparent with Giemsa-stained preparations, while they are typically pale orange in Pap-stained preparations (Fig. 6).

The majority of cysts are benign (C2) and do not require further investigation or treatment if asymptomatic. The finding of 3-dimensional epithelial clusters or true papillary fibrovascular cores reveal the presence of a papillary lesion growing inside the cyst [see Chapter 6, this vol., pp. 41–57]. In this eventuality, the lesion must be considered at least "atypical" (C3) and should be subjected to further investigation or be excised.

Fibrocystic Changes

Introduction/Epidemiology

Fibrocystic changes are a common disorder in premenopausal women occurring in 30% of women between 20 and 50 years of age and consisting of an admixture of cystic spaces, stromal fibrosis, and epithelial proliferation. Fibrocystic disease is thought to represent an exaggerated response of breast tissue to hormonal stimulation and may present clinically as an intermittent sensation of pain and swelling related to the menstrual cycle. Symptoms usually cease 1 or 2 years after the menopause.

There are no specific mammographic abnormalities to recognize this lesion, which might be either detectable as an architectural distortion or indeterminate calcifications or be completely silent. Ultrasound is usually able to distinguish the cystic spaces inside the lesion, but the hypoechoic appearance of the surrounding tissue, together with the indistinct margins, make it a potential target of cytohistological investigation.

Fibrocystic changes are included in the broad category of "nonproliferative" breast lesions. Although the association between nonproliferative disease and cancer is still an unclear and debated issue, it is established that women with nonproliferative disease have a lower risk than those with proliferative disease [Castells et al., 2015; Hartmann et al., 2005].

Histological Features

Breast tissue with fibrocystic changes is characterized by the presence of fibrosclerotic stroma containing cystically dilated ducts that may lack epithelial lining or show apocrine metaplasia. Cyst diameter varies from 1–2 mm to a few centimeters and may be surrounded by inflammatory cells attesting previous ruptures. A certain grade of "usual-type" ductal hyperplasia is frequent. Acinar units are often increased in number, enlarged, and may be lined by columnar cells (Fig. 7).

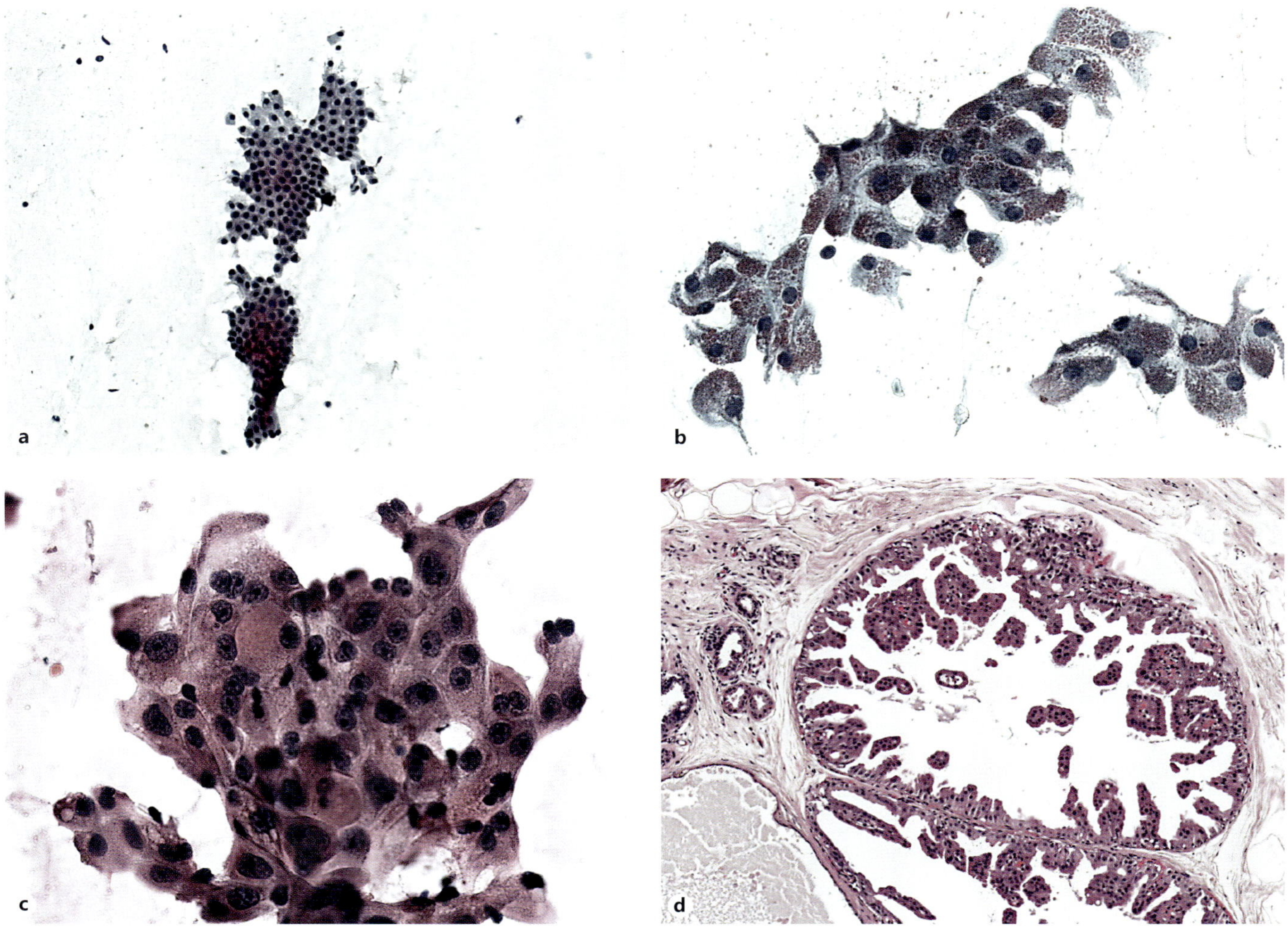

Fig. 5. Apocrine metaplastic cyst. An epithelial component may be present in cystic lesions and might be represented by sheets of apocrine cells (**a**). Apocrine cells show a central round nucleus with a single, small nucleolus, and wide, finely granular cytoplasm (**b**). On H&E-stained preparations, apocrine cells show a distinct granular eosinophilic cytoplasm and may sometimes display some nuclear abnormalities (**c**). The apocrine epithelium lining the cyst frequently produces papillary projections, but this should not be considered as a true papillary lesion (**d**). Papanicolaou (**a**, **b**) and H&E (**c**, **d**). **a** Intermediate power. **b**, **c** High power. **d** Low power.

Cytology

The cytological aspects of fibrocystic changes are many and variable, reflecting the heterogeneous nature of the lesions. The aspired material can be scant and is frequently "watery" in appearance and consistency. The smears show a variable number of histiocytes with foamy cytoplasm, sclerotic stromal fragments, and epithelial cell layers. The epithelial component, if prominent, represents the most worrying aspect of this lesion, being composed of monolayer sheets, sometimes with "finger-like" projections very similar to those of fibroadenomas, as well as hypercellular and 3-dimensional cell clusters, mimicking proliferative breast disease or well-differentiated carcinoma. Pseudopapillary, branching clusters of ductal or apocrine cells may be present, making the differential diagnosis with papillary lesions challenging, but true fibrovascular cores and/or stellate and meshwork fragments are typically absent (Fig. 8, 9). Epithelial cell nuclei are regular and homogeneous, with fine chromatin, and myoepithelial cells are usually evident above ductal cell sheets or in the background as bare bipolar nuclei. Rarely, the aspirated cells may show some slight nuclear atypia [see Chapter 6, this vol., pp. 41–57].

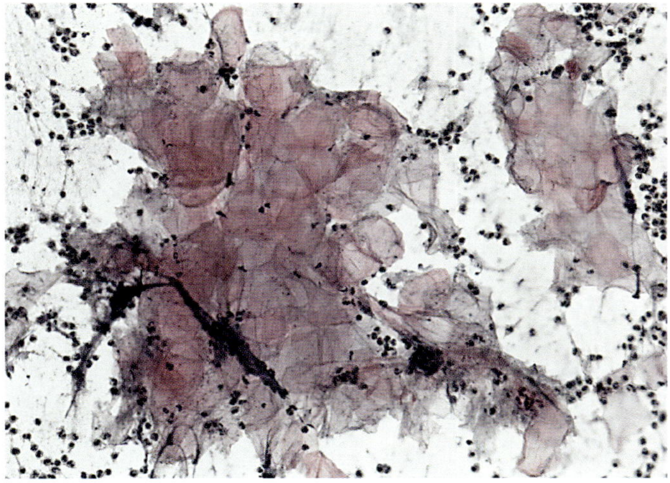

Fig. 6. Epidermal cyst. Keratinocytes with wide pinkish cytoplasm, mainly anucleated (keratin squames), or with a small and pyknotic nucleus are evident in this aspirate. Numerous granulocytes are present as well, indicating an acute inflammatory process. Diagnostic category: C2 (benign). Papanicolaou. High power.

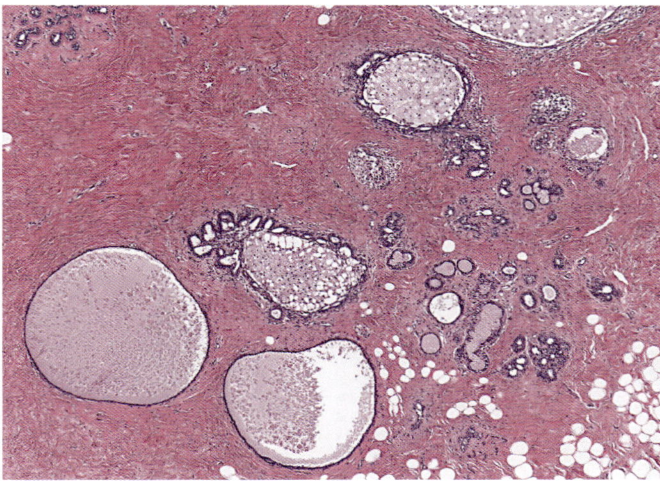

Fig. 7. Histological aspect of fibrocystic changes. The lesion is composed of cystically dilated ducts and acinar structures surrounded by fibrosclerotic stroma. The epithelial component may be hyperplastic and/or show foci of apocrine or columnar cell metaplasia. H&E. Scanning magnification.

Summary

Key Cytological Features of Fibrocystic Changes

- Low to moderate cellularity
- Foamy histiocytes
- Small-sized sheets of benign ductal cells with myoepithelium
- Apocrine cells
- Stromal fragments
- Amorphous, "watery" background

Common Pitfalls of FNA: Fibrocystic Changes

- Three-dimensional epithelial clusters from hyperplastic areas
- Slight cytological atypia

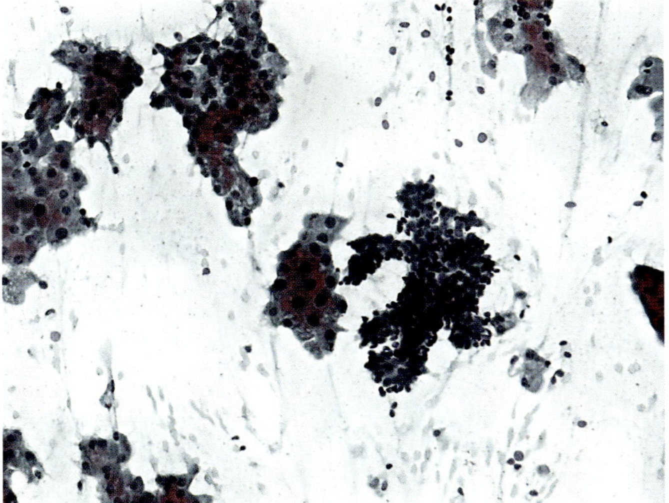

Fig. 8. Cytology of fibrocystic changes. Branching epithelial clusters admixed with apocrine cell layers. Bare bipolar nuclei are visible in the background. Papanicolaou. Intermediate power.

Duct Ectasia

Introduction/Epidemiology

Ectasia of intermediate and major milk ducts is a common occurrence in women of almost any age and is associated with periductal inflammation and fibrosis. Its precise etiology is not known: some authors believe it is caused by glandular atrophy and involution followed by stasis of secretion, leakage of lipid material through the walls, and subsequent periductal inflammation, while others are in favor of a primarily inflammatory cause with subsequent sclerosis and duct dilation. This lesion is suspected in the presence of a spontaneous, intermittent nipple discharge associated or

Fig. 9. Fibrocystic changes. This case was taken from a 35-year-old woman with breast tenderness and several nodules with inhomogeneous structure (hypo- and anechoic) at sonographic examination. The panoramic view of the cytological smear reveals discrete cellularity with wide monolayer epithelial sheets and a watery background (**a**). At higher magnification, small apocrine clusters, stromal fragments, and scattered foamy macrophages are evident (**b–d**). The epithelial cell layers do not show cytological or architectural atypia, while myoepithelial cells, as well as bare bipolar nuclei, are easily identified. Diagnostic category: C2 (benign). Papanicolaou. **a** Scanning magnification. **b** Low power. **c**, **d** Intermediate power.

not with subareolar tissue thickening. Dilated ducts may be palpable and have been described as "wormlike masses." Pain is usually reported among the early symptoms and is more frequent in young women, while the older ones tend to develop nipple inversion or retraction.

Since this lesion develops in the subareolar region, mammography is usually not able to detect it, unless calcifications are present inside dilated ducts. The presence of advanced fibrosis can render the lesion visible as a suspicious stellate opacity. Ultrasound may provide evidence of the ductal dilation inside or upstream of the lesion.

Histological Features

The lesion is composed of one or more dilated ducts surrounded by fibrosclerotic tissue and lymphocytic infiltrate. Ducts are filled with granular secretion including degenerated epithelial cells or histiocytes. Histiocytes with opaque cytoplasm [first described as "pigmented periductal cells" by Davies in 1974] are typically abundant in the stroma around the duct and even inside the epithelial lining (Fig. 10). Squamous metaplasia may be present in the ductal epithelium [Rosen, 2009].

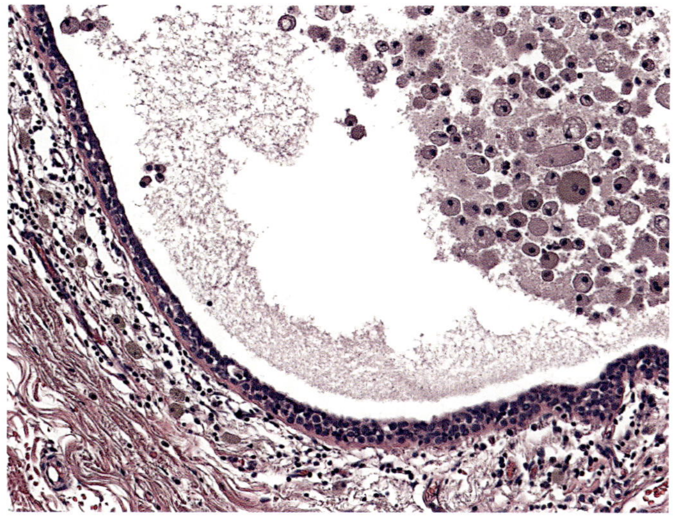

Fig. 10. Histological aspect of duct ectasia. This dilated retroareolar milk duct is filled with proteinaceous secretion and foamy macrophages, which are also present in the stroma right below the epithelial layer, together with some lymphocytes. H&E. Intermediate power.

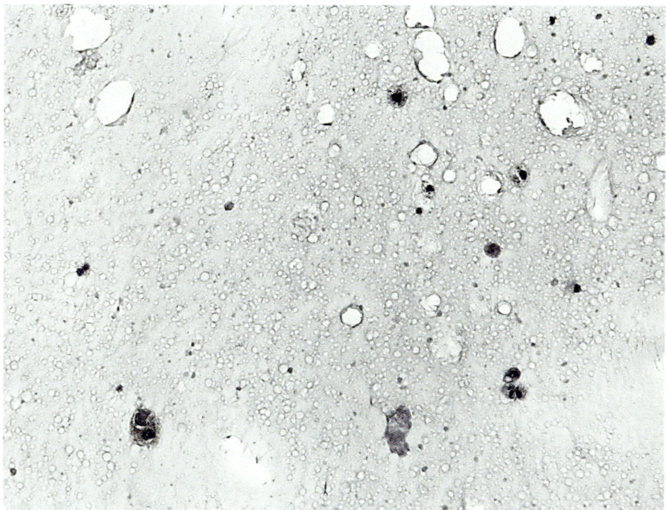

Fig. 11. Duct ectasia. Aspirates or nipple discharge smears taken from duct ectasia are scarcely cellular and display few foamy macrophages and/or degenerated epithelial cells in a watery background. Papanicolaou. Intermediate power.

Cytology

The cytological material may be collected through FNAC or by smearing nipple discharge fluid. This material is usually clear, yellow-green, or brown, and it is usually devoid of epithelial cells, containing a variable number of foamy histiocytes and red blood cells. The background can appear dirty, with abundant granular debris, mucoid, or watery, and some dispersed inflammatory cells are frequently present (Fig. 11).

The extremely scant cellularity of aspirates, which may completely lack epithelial cells, could lead the cytopathologists to consider the examination as unsatisfactory (C1), but in the absence of atypical cells and presence of the key features of watery background and foamy macrophages, and consistent with the sonographic data, a benign diagnosis (C2) can safely be made.

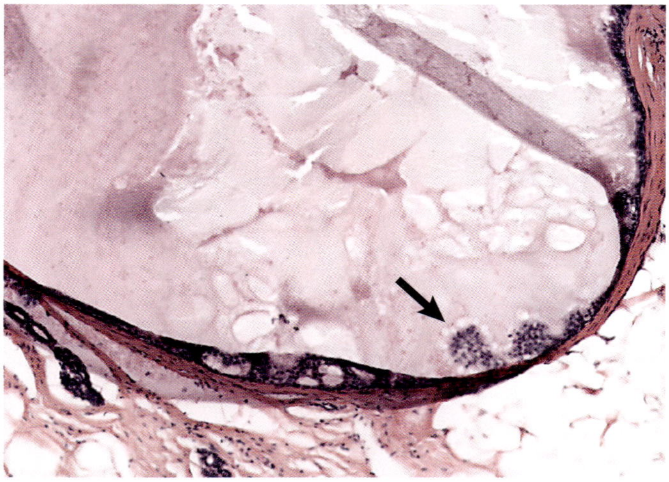

Fig. 12. Histology of a mucocele-like lesion. The lesion is composed of a cystically dilated duct filled with mucin and lined by a variably proliferative epithelium. Small papillary projections are visible in this case (arrow). H&E. Low power.

Mucocele-Like Lesions

Introduction/Epidemiology

Mucocele-like lesions of the breast are composed of distended mucin-filled ducts or cysts lined by a variably hyperplastic ductal epithelium. Once considered benign lesions when first described by Rosen in 1986, they constitute a spectrum ranging from benign to atypical and malignant [Jaffer et al., 2011].

Mucocele-like lesions may be palpable and appear on mammography as well-circumscribed, lobulated masses with or without calcifications [Kim et al., 2005]. Ultrasound shows a hypoechoic, round or lobulated, solid or cystic tumor, sometimes with ill-defined margins.

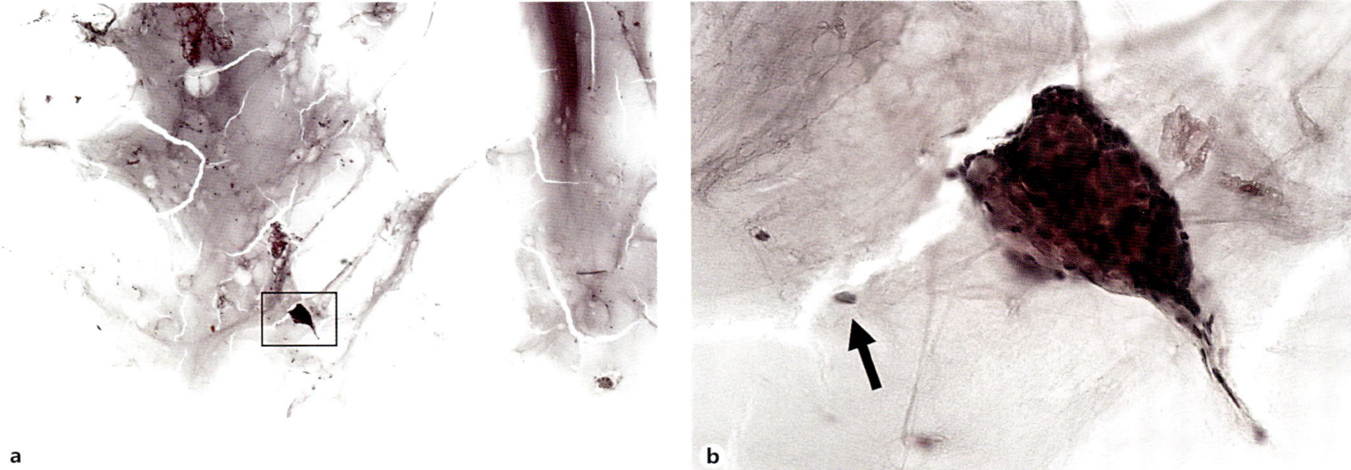

Fig. 13. Cytology of a mucocele-like lesion. The smear is scarcely cellular, almost completely occupied by a homogeneous mucous substance (**a**). Some small epithelial cell clusters are entrapped in the mucus, and scattered bare bipolar nuclei are present in the background (arrow) (**b**). Papanicolaou. **a** Low power. **b** High power.

Histological Features

Histological examination of these lesions shows a cluster of cystically dilated, often ruptured ducts with abundant mucinous secretion discharged into the adjacent stroma. The ducts are lined by a flat or low cuboidal epithelium with occasional papillary projections (Fig. 12). Areas of atypical ductal hyperplasia, as well as ductal carcinoma in situ or invasive mucinous carcinoma might be present. Unlike mucinous carcinoma, benign mucocele-like lesions do not shed epithelial cell clusters "floating" in the mucinous substance [Meares et al., 2016].

Cytology

Aspirates from mucinous lesions are easily recognized due to the presence of abundant mucus in the background, which can be seen as a fine gray to pinkish transparent film or patina in the background on Pap-stained preparations, while it has a typical magenta color in Giemsa-stained preparations. Cellularity may be extremely variable but is more frequently scant or even absent. When epithelial cells are detected in the mucinous material, they typically aggregate in cohesive uniform monolayer sheets (Fig. 13). Myoepithelial cells are evident above ductal cells, and scattered bare bipolar nuclei are typically present in the background. These are extremely important for the differential diagnosis with mucinous carcinoma, which typically lacks myoepithelial cells and bare nuclei. Ductal hyperplasia or ductal carcinoma in situ as an accompanying lesion can be detected in the smear if single cells and mild to moderate cellular atypia are present [see Chapter 6, this vol., pp. 41–57]. These features, as well as the excessive cellularity, should lead the cytopathologist to consider the lesion at least "atypical" (C3) and suggest the need of further investigation or excisional biopsy.

References

Castells X, Domingo L, Corominas JM, Torá-Rocamora I, Quintana MJ, Baré M, Vidal C, Natal C, Sánchez M, Saladié F, Ferrer J, Vernet M, Servitja S, Rodríguez-Arana A, Roman M, Espinàs JA, Sala M: Breast cancer risk after diagnosis by screening mammography of nonproliferative or proliferative benign breast disease: a study from a population-based screening program. Breast Cancer Res Treat 2015;149:237–244.

Davies JD: Pigmented periductal cells (ochrocytes) in mammary dysplasias: their nature and significance. J Pathol 1974;114:205–216.

Hartmann LC, Sellers TA, Frost MH, Lingle WL, Degnim AC, Ghosh K, Vierkant RA, Maloney SD, Pankratz VS, Hillman DW, Suman VJ, Johnson J, Blake C, Tlsty T, Vachon CM, Melton LJ 3rd, Visscher DW: Benign breast disease and the risk of breast cancer. N Engl J Med 2005;353:229–237

Jaffer S, Bleiweiss IJ, Nagi CS: Benign mucocele-like lesions of the breast: revisited. Mod Pathol 2011; 24:683–687.

Kim JY, Han BK, Choe YH, Ko YH: Benign and malignant mucocele-like tumors of the breast: mammographic and sonographic appearances. AJR Am J Roentgenol 2005;185:1310–1316.

Meares AL, Frank RD, Degnim AC, Vierkant RA, Frost MH, Hartmann LC, Winham SJ, Visscher DW: Mucocele-like lesions of the breast: a clinical outcome and histologic analysis of 102 cases. Hum Pathol 2016;49:33–38.

Rosen PP: Non proliferative breast lesions; in Rosen PP (ed): Rosen's Breast Pathology, ed 3. Philadelphia, Lippincott Williams & Wilkins, 2009.

Pinamonti M, Zanconati F: Breast Cytopathology. Assessing the Value of FNAC in the Diagnosis of Breast Lesions.
Monogr Clin Cytol. Basel, Karger, 2018, vol 24, pp 41–57 (DOI: 10.1159/000479767)

Epithelial Proliferative Lesions

Epithelial proliferative lesions of the breast are a heterogeneous group of intraepithelial lesions that includes ductal hyperplasia without atypia, atypical ductal hyperplasia (ADH), low-grade ductal carcinoma in situ (DCIS), glandular adenosis, intraductal papillomas, lobular intraepithelial neoplasia (LIN), and radial scar (RS)/complex sclerosing lesion (CSL). These can be extremely difficult to subclassify on cytological specimens [Sneige and Staerkel, 1994; Frost et al., 1997; Silverman et al., 1993], but a strong effort must be made by cytopathologists to make a distinction between the major categories, especially those requiring different management and treatment. Beyond the direct consequences of a "benign" or a "malignant" diagnosis, the correct identification of proliferative breast lesions is fundamental in predicting the possible subsequent development of invasive carcinoma [Abendroth et al., 1991].

Note that a definite diagnosis of proliferative breast lesions may be difficult also on core needle biopsy and even on a surgical specimen due to the marked interobserver variability and the heterogeneity of the lesions themselves, which may show a mix of coexisting different features [Schnitt et al., 1992]. In this chapter, we give some hints regarding the interpretation of aspirates taken from epithelial proliferative lesions, trying to underline the differences between the main categories in order to guide the patients to the best management.

Ductal Epithelial Hyperplasia

Introduction/Epidemiology

Ductal epithelial hyperplasia without atypia or usual hyperplasia lies at one end of the spectrum of breast proliferative lesions, opposite to high-grade DCIS. It is a common breast alteration, as it is found in approximately 30% of breast biopsies with a benign diagnosis [Lakhani et al., 2012]. It is a nonpalpable lesion and might be detected in the presence of calcifications or be a part of a complex lesion.

Histological Features

Usually, hyperplasia consists of an increase in the number of epithelial cell layers lining the ducts, which may form cellular bridges across the duct lumen. The nuclei have a haphazard orientation and do not show significant irregularities in size, shape, and chromatin pattern (Fig. 1). The histolog-

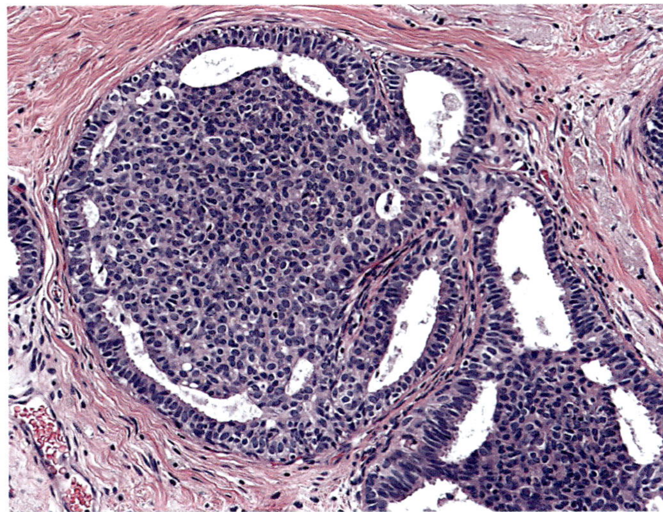

Fig. 1. Histology of usual epithelial hyperplasia. The proliferating ductal epithelial cells form cellular bridges across the lumen. The nuclei have a haphazard orientation and do not show significant irregularities in size, shape, and chromatin pattern. H&E. Low power.

ical definition of this lesion includes the terms *mild* ductal hyperplasia when there are 2 or 4 ductal cell layers, *moderate* hyperplasia when there are more layers, and *florid* hyperplasia when the layers are so numerous to fill the ductal lumen completely. This might determine the formation of secondary, slit-like lumina at the periphery of the duct.

Cytology

Aspirates from areas of ductal hyperplasia without atypia usually display wide monolayer sheets of ductal cells with round to oval nuclei, a discrete amount of cytoplasm, and visible intercellular spaces in a honeycomb structure (Fig. 2). Myoepithelial cells are evident above ductal cells. Some single epithelial cells with intact cytoplasm may be present, mimicking low-grade carcinoma, but these cells do not show significant nuclear atypia: nuclear borders are neat and regular, chromatin is finely dispersed, and nucleoli are small. Epithelial layers may seldom show digit-form projections similar to those seen in aspirates from fibroadenomas (Fig. 3) [see Chapter 7, this vol., pp. 58–67].

Aspirates should be considered benign (C2) if they are mainly composed of cohesive epithelial monolayer sheets with evident myoepithelial cells and without significant atypia, a concept that will be explained in detail in the following paragraphs.

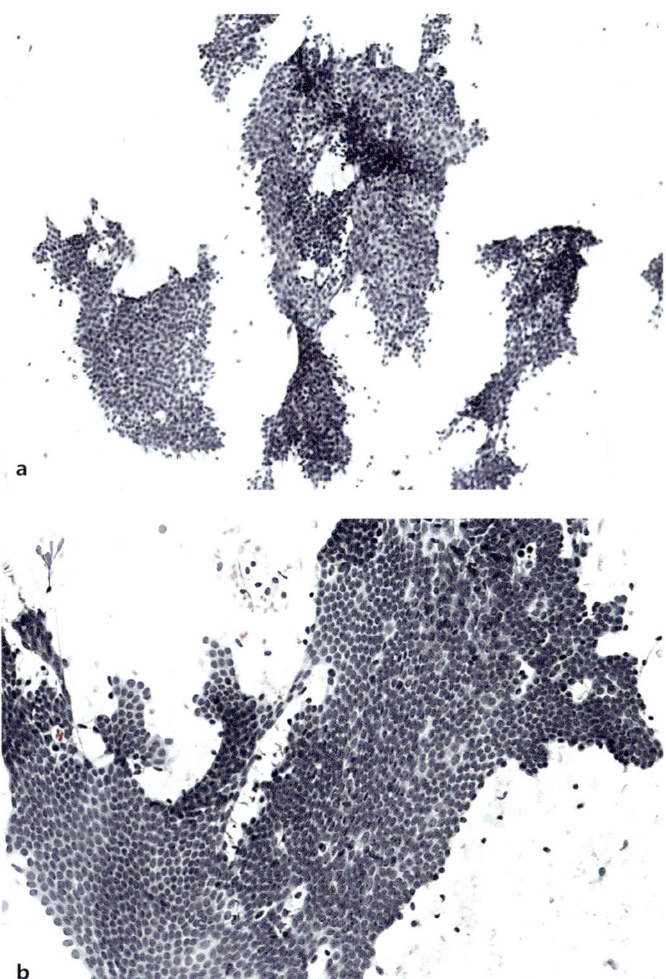

Fig. 2. Cytology of usual epithelial hyperplasia. This smear is highly cellular and is composed mainly of wide monolayer sheets of uniform ductal cells with honeycomb structure and myoepithelial cells. These epithelial layers show focally a cribriform configuration (**b**). Scattered bare nuclei are evident in the background. Papanicolaou. **a** Low power. **b** Intermediate power.

Summary

Key Cytological Features of Ductal Epithelial Hyperplasia

- Moderate to marked cellularity
- Monolayer sheets of ductal cells with myoepithelial cells
- Low to moderate number of isolated epithelial cells
- No cytological atypia

Common Pitfalls of FNA: Ductal Epithelial Hyperplasia

- High number of isolated cells
- Slight nuclear atypia

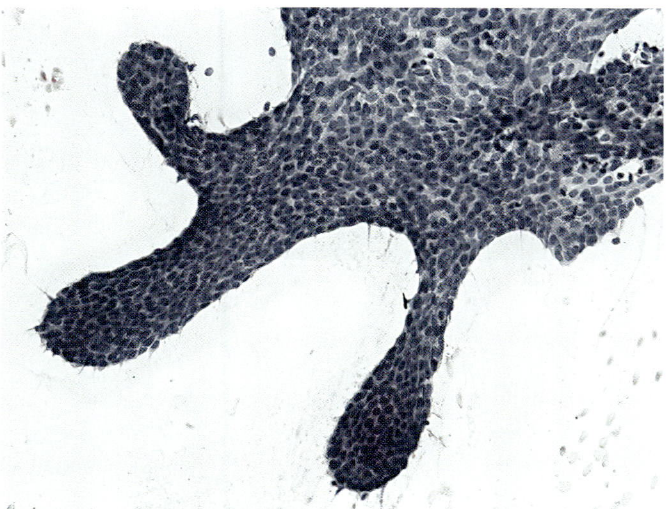

Fig. 3. Usual epithelial hyperplasia. Epithelial cell clusters may form digit-form projections resembling those of fibroadenomas. Note the neat and curved edges of the cluster, presence of myoepithelial cells, and homogeneity of nuclei. Papanicolaou. Intermediate power.

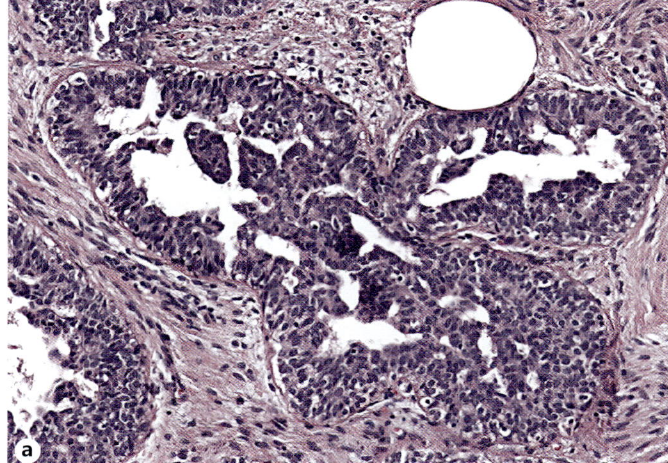

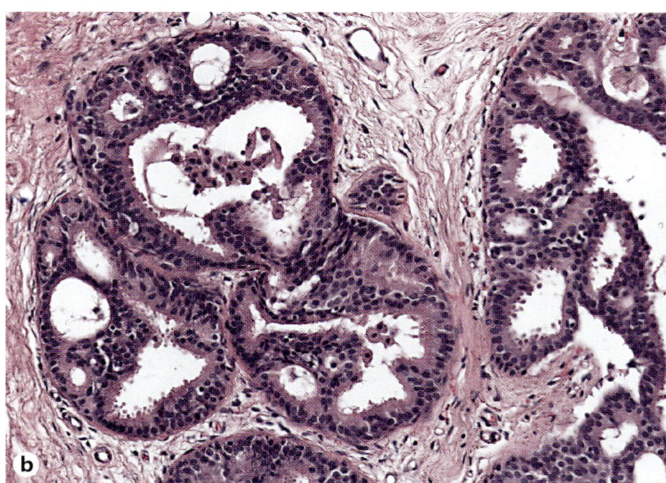

Fig. 4. Histological features of atypical ductal hyperplasia/low-grade ductal carcinoma in situ. Ductal spaces are partially filled with hyperplastic epithelium showing mild nuclear atypia and a micropapillary (**a**) or cribriform (**b**) configuration. The distinction between atypical ductal hyperplasia and low-grade ductal carcinoma in situ is mainly based on dimensions. H&E. Intermediate power.

Atypical Epithelial Hyperplasia and Low-Grade Ductal Carcinoma in situ

Introduction/Epidemiology

ADH and low-grade DCIS represent both close steps in the spectrum of breast epithelial proliferative lesions. They are usually asymptomatic and detected through mammography in the presence of calcifications, which are typically assessed as "indeterminate" by the radiologists, and contrary to the coarse, pleomorphic, and branched ones seen in high-grade DCIS with comedo necrosis. Some low-grade DCIS might be mass forming and present as palpable masses.

DCIS is a heterogeneous disease that can be divided into several subgroups (namely *solid, papillary, cribriform,* and *comedo*) based on its architectural features and into low and high grade based on the degree of nuclear alterations and the presence or absence of necrosis. Low- and high-grade DCISs represent 2 genetically distinct entities, which may lead to the development of different types of invasive breast carcinoma. High-grade lesions have a greater tendency to evolve into invasive cancer (usually high-grade histotypes), they are easy to recognize as malignant lesions on aspirates as well as core biopsies, and the main differential diagnosis includes invasive cancer. Conversely, low-grade DCIS is an indolent and slowly progressing lesion that may evolve into well-differentiated invasive carcinomas [Simpson et al., 2005].

We defer the discussion on high-grade DCIS to Chapter 8 [this vol., pp. 68–93]; its cytological findings are very similar to those of invasive breast carcinoma.

Histological Features

ADH and low-grade DCIS present histologically as monotonous epithelial ductal proliferations with a solid, micro-

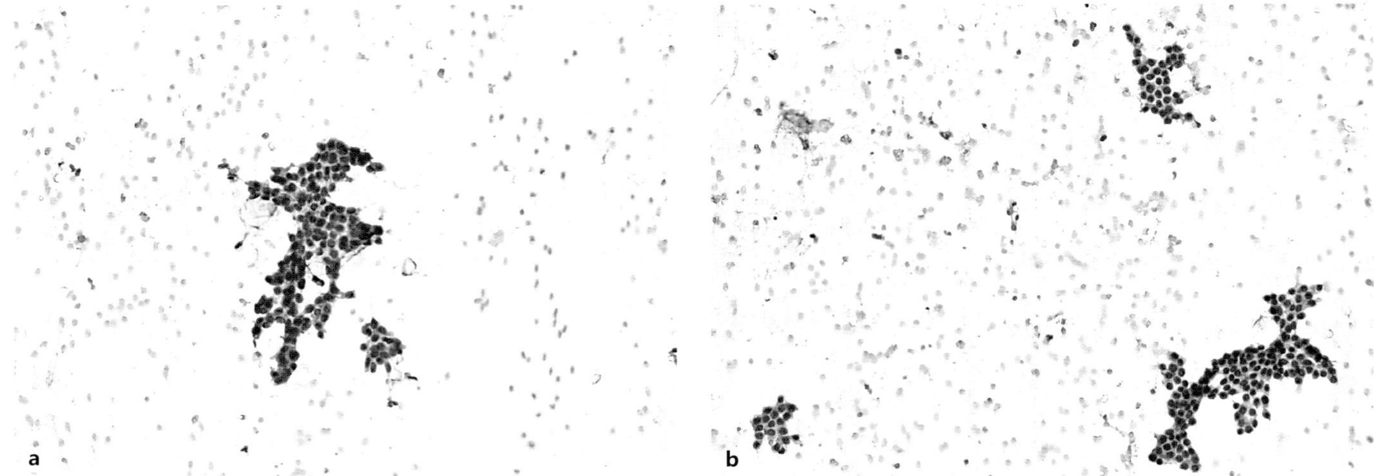

Fig. 5. Epithelial hyperplasia with mild atypia. Cellularity in this smear is composed of monolayer or slightly hyperplastic clusters of rather uniform epithelial cells. These are not the broad sheets with honeycomb structure of a completely benign-looking proliferation and show slight architectural complexity (**a**, **b**). Some clusters lack myoepithelial cells. This lesion was prudently assessed as "undetermined, probably benign" (C3) and close follow-up was recommended. Papanicolaou. **a**, **b** Intermediate power.

papillary, or cribriform architecture lacking necrosis or with only small foci of necrosis and without severe nuclear atypia (Fig. 4). The distinction between ADH and low-grade DCIS is mainly based on their dimensions or quantitative characteristics [Lakhani et al., 2012] and thus cannot be assessed on cytological specimens.

Cytology

The diagnosis of atypia in breast FNAC is a source of controversy between cytopathologists [Lim et al., 2004]. It includes nuclear atypia and/or architectural atypia (poor cellular cohesiveness and complexity and branching of tissue fragments) [Dawson et al., 1995; Sneige and Staerkel, 1994].

Aspirates taken from ADH or low-grade DCIS show moderately to highly cellular epithelial layers, which may show a cribriform or papillary architecture, solid 3-dimensional aggregates, and a discrete number of isolated intact epithelial cells. Epithelial cell nuclei are usually 1.5–2 times the size of a red blood cell and may show some slight irregularity in size, shape, or chromatin pattern but are generally monotonous. The smears typically display an admixture of normal benign epithelial fragments and atypical clusters (Fig. 5–7) [Shin and Sneige, 1998].

The presence of such characteristics is usually sufficient to enter the case in the category of undetermined (C3) or suspicious lesions (C4), which need further diagnostic investigation through a tissue biopsy.

The presence of many dispersed cells with high-grade nuclear abnormalities and an inflammatory background raises the possibility of a high-grade comedo DCIS or a high-grade invasive carcinoma. Cytology is unable to make an accurate distinction between in situ and invasive carcinoma, also because they are frequently found in association to each other. Thus, the finding of high-grade malignant cells must lead the pathologist to consider the lesion as malignant and immediately address the patient to the adequate treatment.

Summary

Key Cytological Features of Atypical Ductal Hyperplasia/Low-Grade Ductal Carcinoma in situ

- Moderate to marked cellularity
- Variable number of single dissociated cells
- Some 3-dimensional clusters and epithelial layers with pseudopapillary and/or cribriform arrangement
- Slight nuclear abnormalities (shape, size, and chromatin distribution)
- Admixture of benign and atypical cell layers

Lobular Intraepithelial Neoplasia

Introduction/Epidemiology

The term lobular intraepithelial neoplasia includes lesions defined as atypical lobular neoplasia and lobular carcinoma

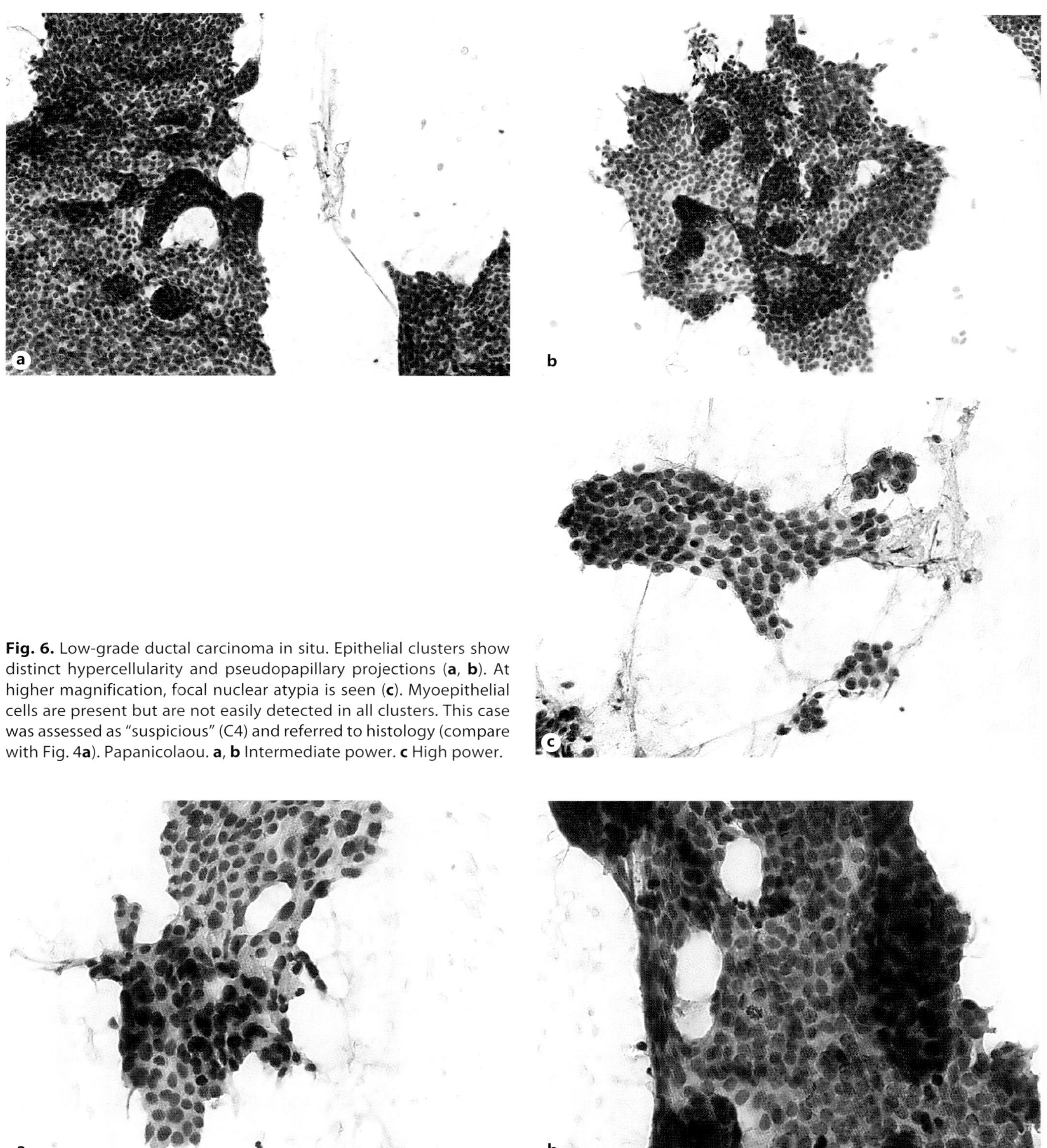

Fig. 6. Low-grade ductal carcinoma in situ. Epithelial clusters show distinct hypercellularity and pseudopapillary projections (**a**, **b**). At higher magnification, focal nuclear atypia is seen (**c**). Myoepithelial cells are present but are not easily detected in all clusters. This case was assessed as "suspicious" (C4) and referred to histology (compare with Fig. 4**a**). Papanicolaou. **a**, **b** Intermediate power. **c** High power.

Fig. 7. Low-grade ductal carcinoma in situ. In this case, atypia is expressed by slight irregularities in nuclear size and shape (**a**) and mitotic activity (**b**). This lesion was diagnosed as suspicious (C4) and subjected to core needle biopsy, with histological confirmation of low-grade ductal carcinoma in situ. Papanicolaou. High power.

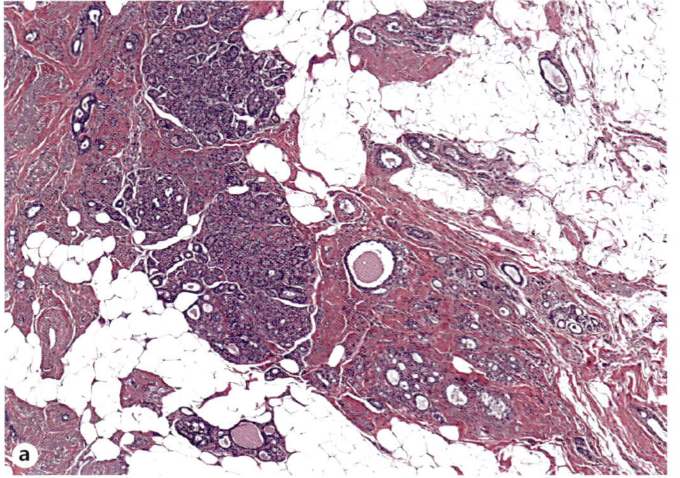

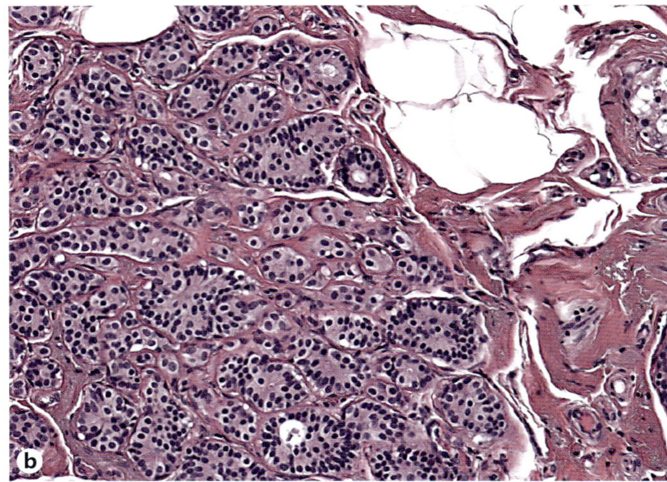

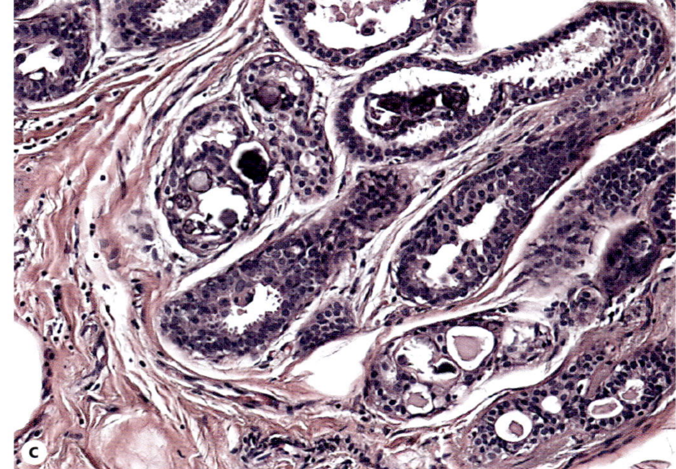

Fig. 8. Histological features of sclerosing adenosis. Sclerosing adenosis is a complex histologic lesion characterized by expansion of the terminal ductal lobular units and fibrosis of the intralobular stroma. The lesion might show a pseudo-infiltrative growth pattern that renders its sonographic findings suspicious. The stromal fibrosis and epithelial proliferation might obliterate the small duct lumina and produce microcalcifications (**c**). H&E. **a** Scanning magnification. **b**, **c** Intermediate power.

in situ, which are distinguished based on quantitative criteria [Lakhani et al., 2012]. LIN is typically asymptomatic; unlike DCIS, it does not produce calcifications, even remains undetected by high-resolution radiological techniques, and is most of the time an incidental finding in breast biopsies performed for other reasons. It is reported in approximately 0.5–4% of otherwise benign breast biopsies, but its true incidence is largely unknown. LIN is considered a risk factor for the development of invasive breast carcinoma of either ductal or lobular type in either breast [Ellis et al., 2003].

Because of the difficulty in identifying LIN through mammography and ultrasound, the frequent multicentricity and bilaterality of the lesion, and its unpredictable behavior, the management of patients diagnosed with LIN on biopsy is still a highly debated topic. Some authors recommend excisional biopsy when a focal lesion can be identified, since on surgical excision LIN is associated with a more serious lesion in a significant number of cases [Elsheikh and Silverman, 2005; Purdie et al., 2010], while others advocate close follow-up and recommend excision only when radiology/pathology discordance is found [Nagi et al., 2008].

Histological Features

LIN is characterized by the presence of a uniform population of small, round-shaped, monomorphic cells filling the acini with obliteration of the acinar lumina and possible extension to the adjacent ductal epithelium with a *pagetoid* pattern. These small cells typically do not show significant atypia, with the exception of the pleomorphic variant, and lack the immunohistochemical expression of E-cadherin.

Fig. 9. Cytology of sclerosing adenosis. Cellularity of aspirates taken from sclerosing adenosis can vary widely and is moderate in this case, with many epithelial cell clusters of different shapes and sizes (**a**). At higher magnification, these clusters are slightly hypercellular and have tubular or acinar configuration, with evident myoepithelial cells on the surface (**b**, **c**). Additional findings include sclerotic stromal fragments (**c**), scattered bare nuclei, and foamy cells in the background (**d**). Papanicolaou. **a** Scanning magnification. **b–d** Intermediate power.

Cytology

LIN is rarely encountered in FNAC, since it is not palpable and not detected by ultrasound. Nevertheless, it might occur adjacent to or in the context of another lesion and present in the aspirate as an occasional finding. It displays a variable number of uniform, small cells with bland, eccentric nuclei and vacuolated cytoplasm, arranged singly or in tight clusters.

The main differential diagnosis to be considered is invasive lobular carcinoma, which is made up of the same cells, and, in such cases, the radiological features of the lesion are helpful. Since LIN is asymptomatic and neither visualized by ultrasound nor by mammography, features of the original lesion that lead to a biopsy should be present in the aspirate.

Adenosis and Sclerosing Adenosis

Introduction/Epidemiology

"Adenosis" is a term used to define an increment in the number of acinar structures in breast lobules. Sclerosing adenosis is a distinct lesion characterized by the architectural disorganization of the terminal ductal-lobular unit with epithelial and myo-

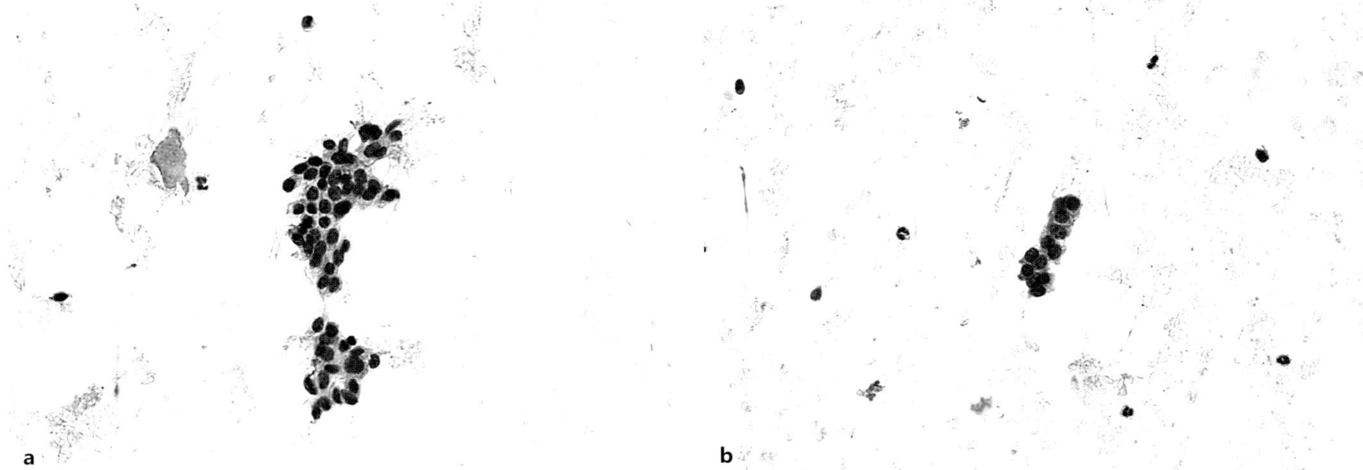

Fig. 10. Sclerosing adenosis. This smear is loosely cellular and has scattered, small epithelial cell clusters without significant cytological atypia (**a**). Myoepithelial cells are rare or even absent in some clusters, and this finding, together with the poor cell-to-cell cohesion and the occasional single cells (**b**), was sufficient to put this case in the suspicious category (C4). On histological evaluation, it turned out to be an area of sclerosing adenosis. Papanicolaou. **a**, **b** High power.

epithelial proliferation and stromal fibrosis [Jensen et al., 1989], a well-known source of diagnostic errors [Cho and Oh, 2001; Sreedharanunni et al., 2013]. It is a common finding, which occurs in 27.8% of all benign biopsies, and it is associated with an increased risk of invasive breast cancer [Visscher et al., 2014].

Histological Features

The histological examination of sclerosing adenosis shows expansion of the terminal ductal-lobular unit with increased numbers of small-sized acini and dense fibrosis of the intralobular stroma. Stromal fibrosis may compress the glands and obliterate ductal lumina, generating calcifications and giving the lesion a pseudo-invasive appearance (Fig. 8). The presence of myoepithelial cells is the most important clue to recognize this lesion and distinguish it from invasive carcinoma.

Cytology

The presence of irregular calcifications and architectural distortion in sclerosing adenosis may lead to diagnostic biopsies of masses suspicious of an invasive carcinoma. FNAC samples taken from areas of sclerosing adenosis are usually moderately cellular and display many small groups or acinar sheets of uniform ductal cells with myoepithelial cells and bare bipolar nuclei and some hyalinized stromal fragments in the background (Fig. 9). Focal apocrine metaplasia, foamy cells, and scattered individual epithelial cells might be present [Cho and Oh, 2001; Silverman et al., 1989]. The cellularity of the smear and the presence of 3-dimensional clusters, as well as the presence of slight to moderate nuclear pleomorphism, can be misleading and result in false-positive results (Fig. 10). For this reason, much attention should be given to the myoepithelial cells above the epithelial cells and to the presence of bare nuclei.

Possible differential diagnoses include fibroadenoma, which typically shows high cellularity and an admixture of epithelial and stromal fragments. The key elements for this differential diagnosis are the acinar epithelial sheets typical of adenosis rather than in digit form or staghorn clusters of fibroadenoma, the presence of single epithelial cells, and the hyalinized stroma of sclerosing adenosis, which is different from the fibromyxoid one of fibroadenoma (Fig. 11) [Sreedharanunni et al., 2013].

Summary

Key Cytological Features of Sclerosing Adenosis
- Moderate to marked cellularity
- Small acinar and tubular clusters
- Myoepithelial cells and scattered bare nuclei
- Hyalinized stromal fragments

Common Pitfalls of FNA: Sclerosing Adenosis
- Three-dimensional clusters
- Epithelial dissociated cells
- Slight to moderate nuclear pleomorphism

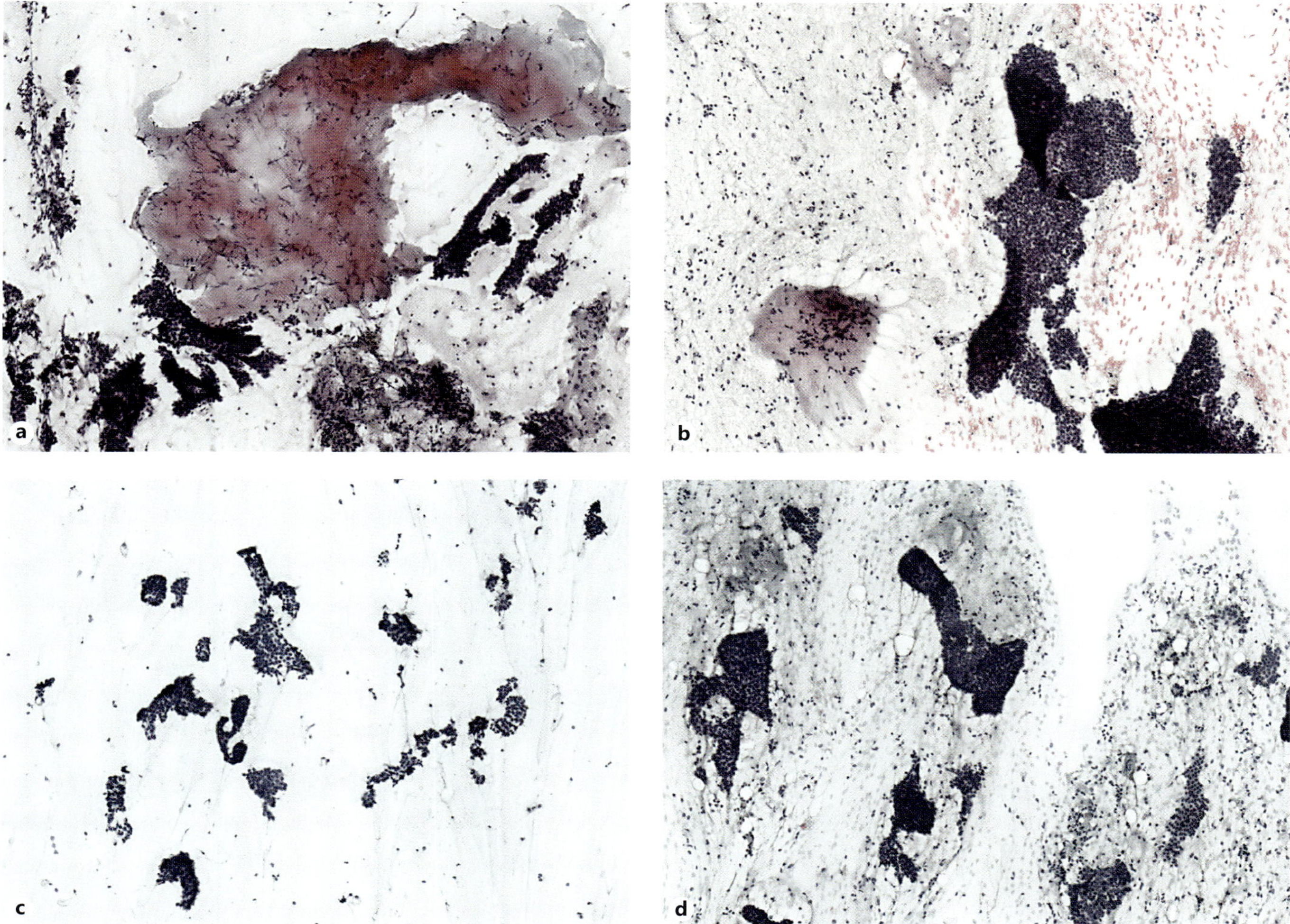

Fig. 11. Comparison between sclerosing adenosis and fibroadenoma. Sclerosing adenosis and fibroadenoma may look very similar to each other on the cytological smear, but a distinction can be made in most cases relying mainly on their different pattern at low magnification. Epithelial clusters of sclerosing adenosis (**a**, **c**) vary widely in size within the same lesion but are usually rather small, and typically they have a distinct tubular or acinar configuration. Conversely, epithelial clusters of fibroadenomas (**b**, **d**) tend to be larger, broader, and show neat round (digit-form) edges. Bare bipolar nuclei are extremely numerous in many fibroadenomas. Furthermore, stromal fragments are sclerotic and hyalinized in sclerosing adenosis, while they are typically myxoid or densely cellular in fibroadenomas. Papanicolaou. Low power.

Intraductal Papilloma (Benign Papillary Lesions of the Breast)

Introduction/Epidemiology

Intraductal papillary lesions of the breast form a wide spectrum of pathological changes, with benign intraductal papilloma on one end of the spectrum and papillary carcinoma at the other end. Papillary lesions may be solitary or multiple, central or peripheral; clinically, they may present as palpable masses or cause nipple discharge (sometimes hematic). Mammography may show well-circumscribed, single, or multiple lesions of varying size with or without calcification. Ultrasound of these lesions may show a complex intracystic lesion or a homogenous solid lesion, often accompanied by duct dilatation [Ganosan et al., 2006].

Histological Features

Intraductal papillary lesions, whether benign or malignant, are characterized by the presence of fibrovascular cores lined by epithelial proliferation with varying degrees of

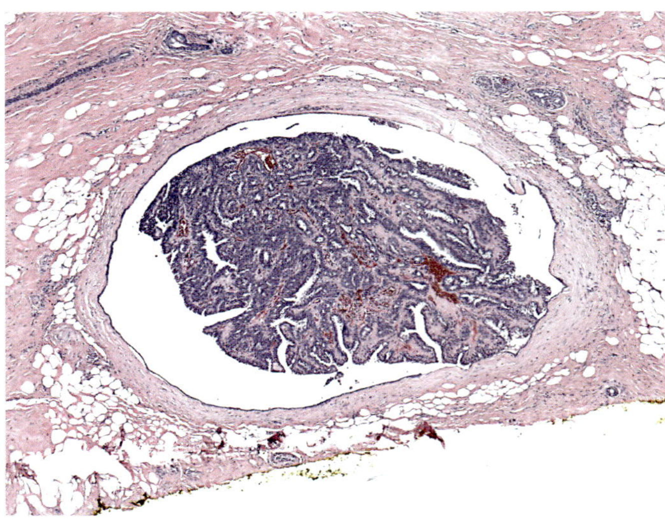

Fig. 12. Intraductal papilloma. This cystically dilated milk duct hosts a papillary lesion composed of a branching fibrovascular stalk lined by uniform columnar epithelial cells without atypia. H&E. Low power.

atypia (Fig. 12). Papillomas may vary in size from less than 1 mm to several centimeters; larger lesions may contain necrotic or hemorrhagic areas and microcalcifications and usually develop inside a dilated duct or a cyst. Ductal epithelial hyperplasia as well as apocrine metaplasia and even cytological atypia may coexist.

Cytology

Many different breast lesions may show "papillary" features on cytological preparations. These include true papillomas and other entities with papillary component, such as RS, fibrocystic change, fibroadenomas, and ductal carcinoma, both in situ and invasive. Though a definite diagnosis of the nature of papillary lesions is possible on an excision biopsy, the distinction is not easy on aspiration cytology. This is due to the overlapping cytological features between benign and malignant as well as other entities containing a papillary component [Simsir et al., 2003].

Cytological smears from intraductal papillomas show moderate to marked cellularity, with abundant isolated columnar cells and 3-dimensional, branched epithelial cell sheets. Tissue fragments are predominantly large, with some scattered smaller fragments (Fig. 13, 14, 16) [Field and Mak, 2006]. Fibrovascular cores are often (but not always) recognizable, as well as dispersed bare nuclei and cyst macrophages [Jeffry and Ljung, 1994]. Field and Mak [2006] emphasized the importance of a clear terminology while describing the so-called "papillary clusters" or "papillary features" in aspirates from breast lesions. They described "stellate" and "meshwork" tissue fragments as highly sensitive and specific morphological features for the diagnosis of intraductal papillomas (Fig. 14).

Papillary lesions might display some features of suspicion in the form of complex papillae and single atypical cells, making the distinction from carcinoma difficult [Reid-Nicholson et al., 2006]. Infarcted papillomas may show moderate atypia, usually associated to hemosiderin-laden macrophages (Fig. 15). Apocrine metaplastic cells with large, granular cytoplasm and round nuclei with small nucleoli are a common finding in papillary lesions. Note that apocrine cell sheets typically do not show myoepithelial cells, and this should not be interpreted as a malignant feature. Some authors suggest that stromal bare nuclei and nuclear atypia may be useful in distinguishing benign from malignant papillary lesions [Nayar et al., 2001]. However, the lack of specificity and sensitivity of these features makes a definite diagnosis of benign papilloma impossible on aspiration cytology. The diagnostic category for such lesions should always be at least "indeterminate, probably benign" (C3), suggesting the need of a close follow-up or surgical excision when cytological-radiological discordance occurs or additional risk factors are present.

Summary

Key Cytological Features of Intraductal Papilloma

- Moderate to marked cellularity
- Predominance of large tissue fragments with scattered small tissue fragments
- Proteinaceous background with macrophages and/or siderophages
- Dissociated columnar cells
- Stellate tissue fragments
- Myoepithelial cells in epithelial cell layers
- Fibrovascular cores
- Apocrine cell sheets

Common Pitfalls of FNA: Intraductal Papilloma

- Cellular atypia
- Lack of myoepithelial cells
- Necrotic or hemorrhagic background

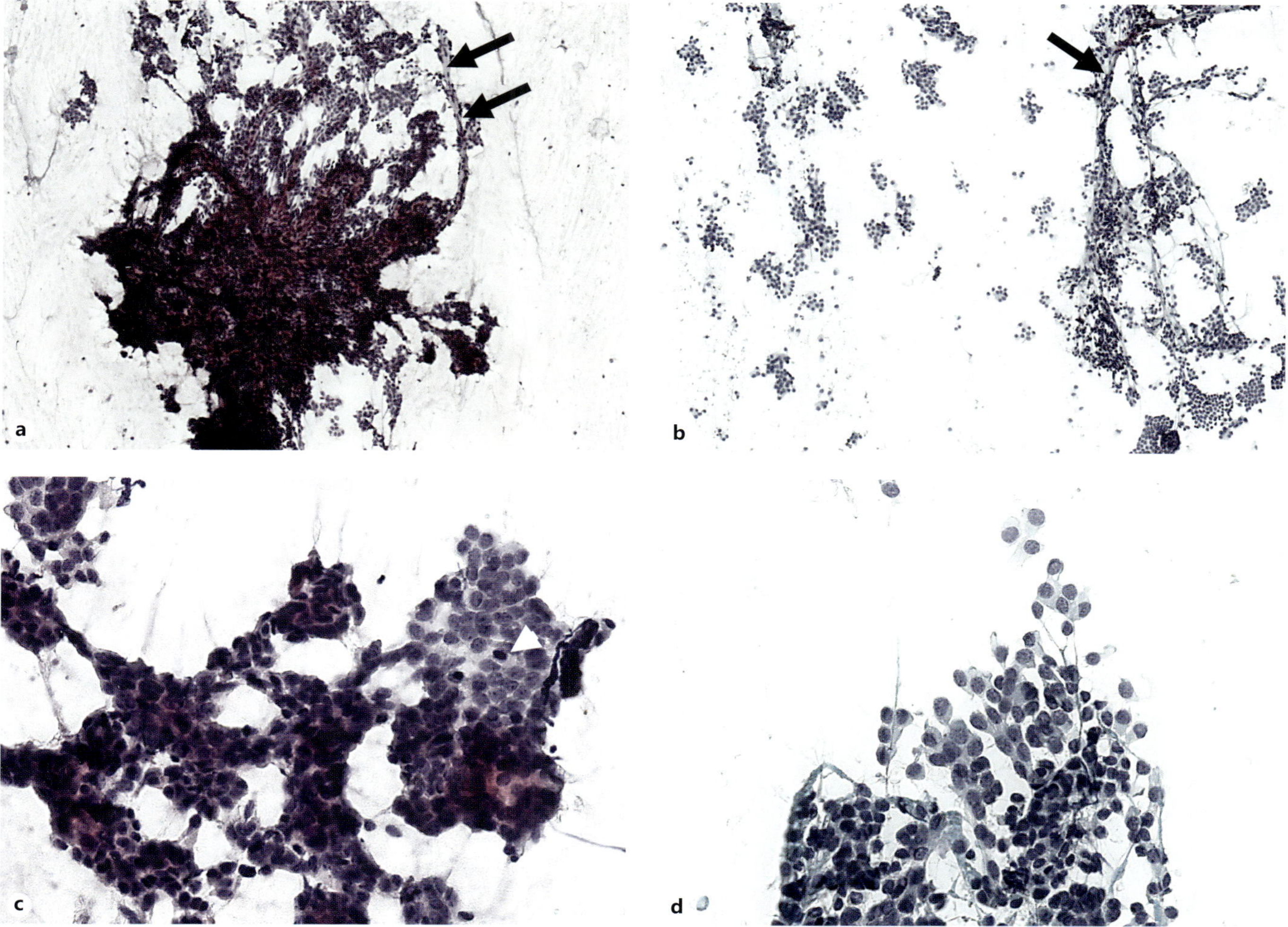

Fig. 13. Cytological features of benign papillary lesions. Aspirates from papillary breast lesions tend to be markedly cellular and show an admixture or large and small epithelial clusters with at least some tendency towards the loss of cell-to-cell cohesion. Larger tissue fragments are often 3-dimensional and branching, and a stromal fibrovascular core may be present (arrows) (**a**, **b**). At higher magnification, attention must be paid to nuclear features and the presence of myoepithelial cells (arrowhead) (**c**). Because of their unpredictable behavior, papillary lesions are never to be considered completely benign, and even those lesions without cytological atypia should be put in the undetermined category (C3). Papanicolaou. **a**, **b** Low power. **c**, **d** High power.

Radial Scar/Complex Sclerosing Lesion

Introduction/Epidemiology

RS is a well-defined radiological and histopathological entity, characterized by a central fibroelastotic core and radiating bands of fibrous tissue containing varying degrees of epithelial proliferation, which can simulate cancer both macroscopically and on microscopic examination [Page and Anderson, 1987]. Lesions larger than 1 cm are defined as CSL. They might be considered as an accentuation of fibrocystic changes associated with epithelial hyperplasia, adenosis, and papillomatosis. The lesion is by definition nonpalpable, and its detection is an incidental finding in 0.09% screening mammograms as a stellate opacity with thin and asymmetric spikes, radiolucent nucleus, and microcalcifications resembling a malignant lesion [Finlay et al., 1994; Loane, 2009].

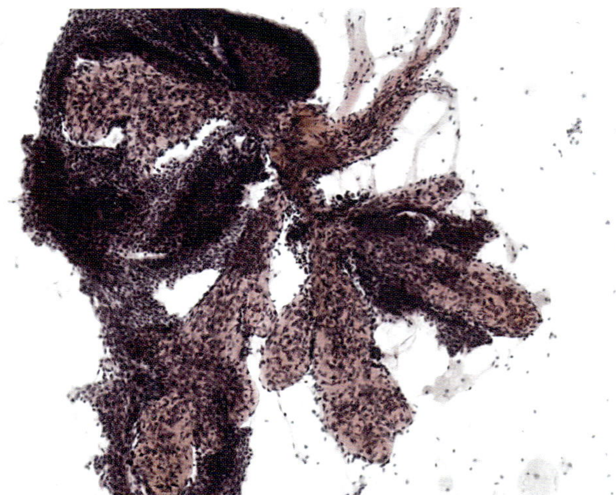

Fig. 14. Intraductal papilloma. The so-called "stellate" tissue fragments are regarded as a highly sensitive and specific morphological feature to correctly diagnose benign papillary lesions of the breast, since they are uncommon in other benign proliferative lesions as well as in papillary carcinomas. Papanicolaou. Low power.

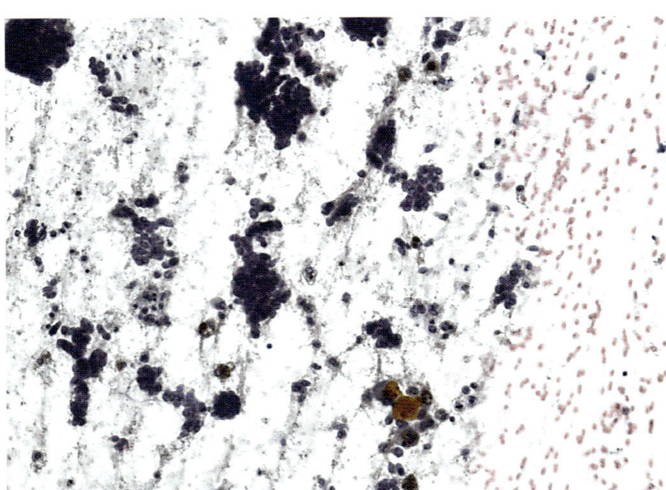

Fig. 15. Infarcted papilloma. The smear is highly cellular and some macrophages with hemosiderin granules in the cytoplasm lie between epithelial cell clusters. Many erythrocytes and granular proteinaceous material are present in the background. Papanicolaou. Intermediate power.

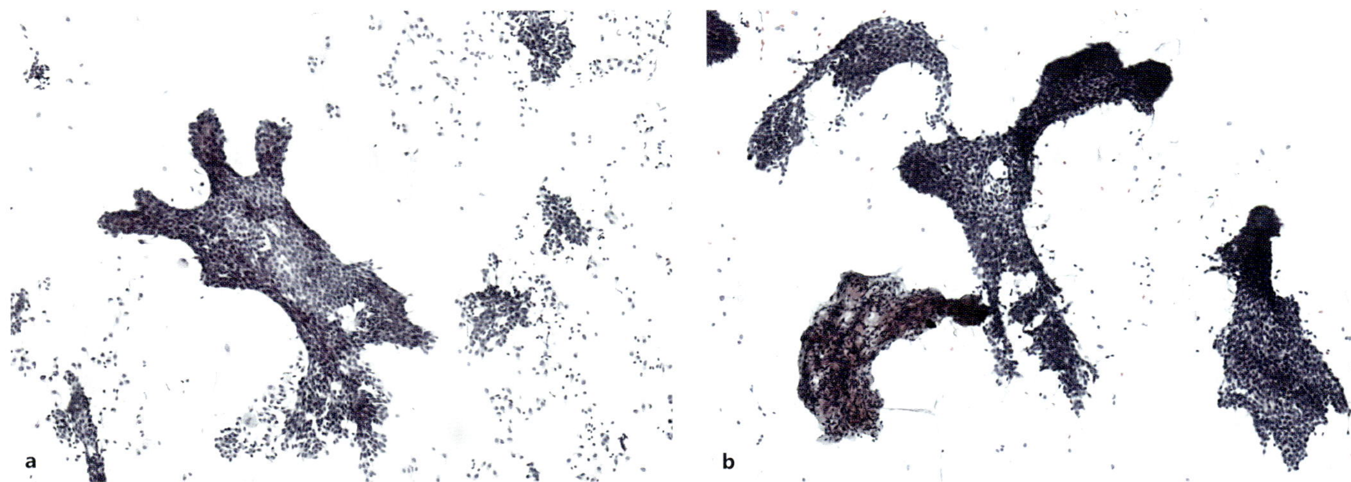

Fig. 16. Comparison between intraductal papilloma and fibroadenoma. Papillary projections of hypercellular epithelial layers in papillary lesions (**a**) may mimic the staghorn epithelial clusters of fibroadenomas (**b**). This resemblance is stronger when fibrovascular cores are not clearly visible in the papillary clusters, as it is in this case. Close examination of the papillary projections may reveal that cells tend to separate from each other, differently from those in the digit-form edges of cell clusters in fibroadenomas. Furthermore, papillary lesions tend to disperse single cells with columnar morphology and intact cytoplasm. Papanicolaou. Low power.

RS/CSL has been found in association with atypical epithelial hyperplasia and ductal carcinoma (both in situ and invasive) [Sloane and Mayers, 1993], and some authors consider it as an independent, increased risk marker for the development of subsequent breast cancer [King et al., 2000].

Histological Features

Histological examination of RS/CSL reveals a central fibroelastotic core with many entrapped small ducts displaying varying degrees of hyperplasia, papillomatosis, apocrine metaplasia, and calcification (Fig. 17). At the periphery of the lesion, normal-looking breast lobules are typically seen.

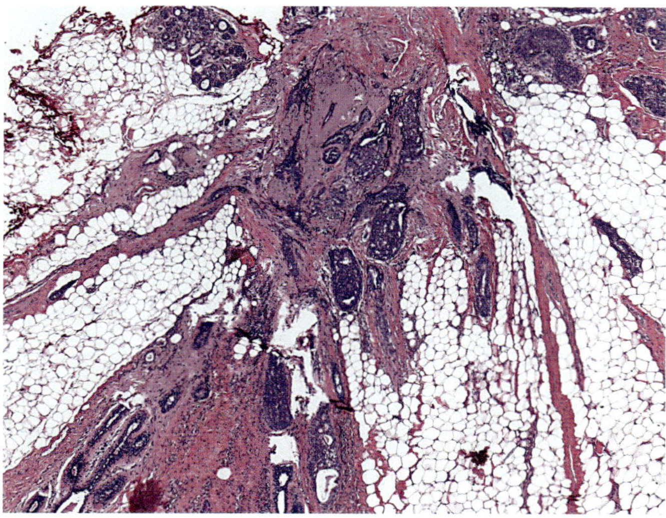

Fig. 17. Histology of radial scar/complex sclerosing lesion. This lesion is composed of a central fibroelastotic core from which many small ducts branch displaying varying degrees of epithelial hyperplasia. H&E. Scanning magnification.

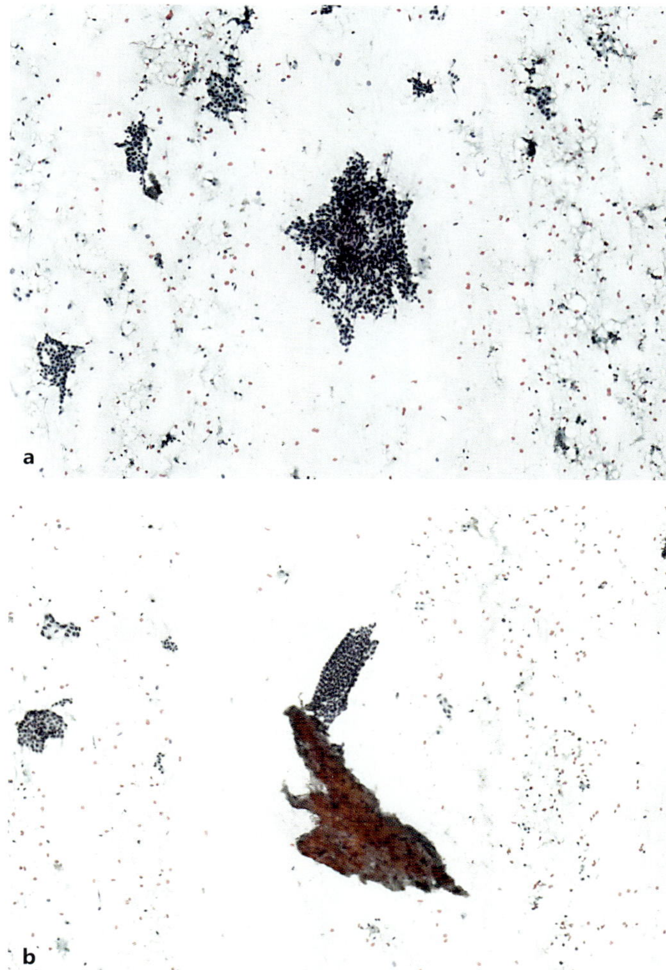

Fig. 18. Cytology of radial scar/complex sclerosing lesion. Aspirates from this kind of lesion usually show moderate to marked cellularity displaying many epithelial monolayer sheets which can have a tubular architecture (**b**). Bare nuclei and fibrillary stromal fragments are present in the background. These lesions are frequently the source of cytoradiological discrepancy. Papanicolaou. **a**, **b** Low power.

CSL are typically heterogeneous, and, in a variable percentage of ADH cases, DCIS and invasive carcinoma may be present within or adjacent to the lesion. For this reason, some authors discourage the use of FNAC or core biopsy alone to make a definite diagnosis and stress the need of a complete excision, especially in lesions larger than 1 cm [King et al., 2000; Nassar et al., 2015].

Cytology

FNAC is generally able to distinguish RS/CSL from a malignant lesion, although the discordance with radiological findings, the various degrees of cytological atypia, and the awareness of having to deal with a heterogeneous and complex lesion should lead to consider a histological excisional approach.

The cytological smear is often moderately to highly cellular with an admixture of large monolayered epithelial sheets and small tubular or acinar clusters with myoepithelial cells and bare bipolar nuclei in the background (Fig. 18). Small papillary clusters, apocrine cells, microcalcifications, and foamy cells are variably present. Typical cytological findings are multiple fibrillary aggregates exhibiting a green tinge on Papanicolaou-stained preparations, representing elastotic material [Bonzanini et al., 1997]. Meshwork and stellate tissue fragments may be present, but are generally less prominent than in papillomas [Field and Mak, 2006].

Prominent nucleoli, scarce cohesiveness, and lack of myoepithelial cells represent the major pitfalls that can pose the suspicion of a malignant lesion. In such cases, the lesion must be considered atypical (C3) or suspicious (C4), and should undergo biopsy for a histological confirmation. Conversely, in cases where cytological atypia is not found in the subsequent core biopsy, some authors suggest that radiological follow-up should be preferred to complete excision [Conlon et al., 2015].

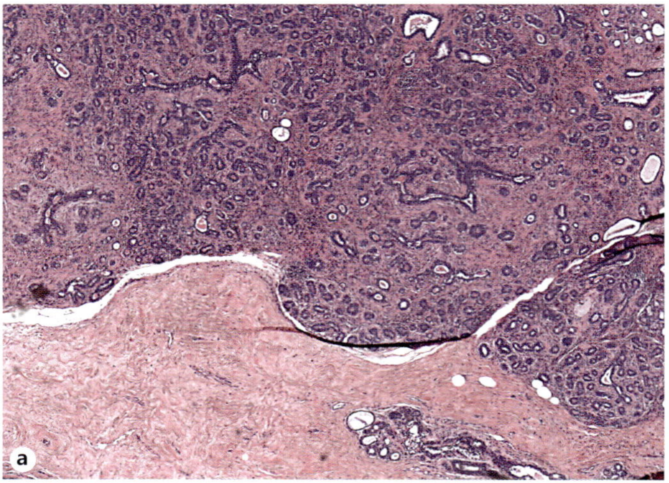
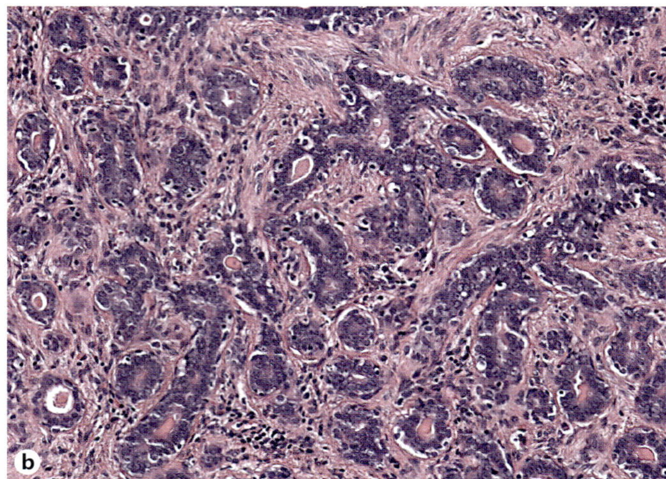

Fig. 19. Histology of tubular adenoma. Tubular adenoma is a nodular mass with neat borders composed of closely packed terminal ducts and acini immersed in a dense, fibrillary intralobular stroma, which, unlike that of fibroadenomas, is not prominent. Epithelial cells do not show significant atypia, and myoepithelial cells are easily detected. H&E. **a** Scanning magnification. **b** Intermediate power.

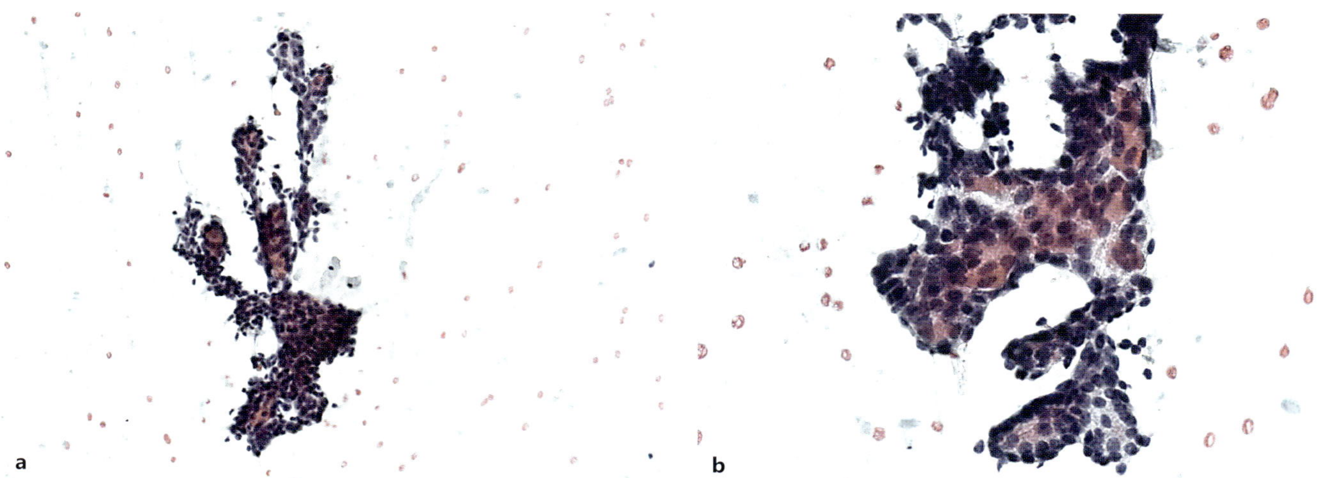

Fig. 20. Cytology of tubular adenoma. Small-sized, branching epithelial clusters with acinar configuration are present in this smear. Epithelial aggregates contain myoepithelial cells, but only occasionally scattered bipolar bare nuclei are present in the background. Papanicolaou. **a** Intermediate power. **b** High power.

Summary

Key Cytological Features of Radial Scar/Complex Sclerosing Lesion

- Moderate to marked cellularity
- Large epithelial honeycomb sheets
- Small tubular and acinar clusters
- Myoepithelial cells
- Papillary or stellate/meshwork tissue fragments
- Fibrillary aggregates

Common Pitfalls of FNA: Radial Scar/Complex Sclerosing Lesion

- Cytological atypia
- Loose cellular cohesiveness
- Lack of myoepithelial cells
- High radiological suspicion

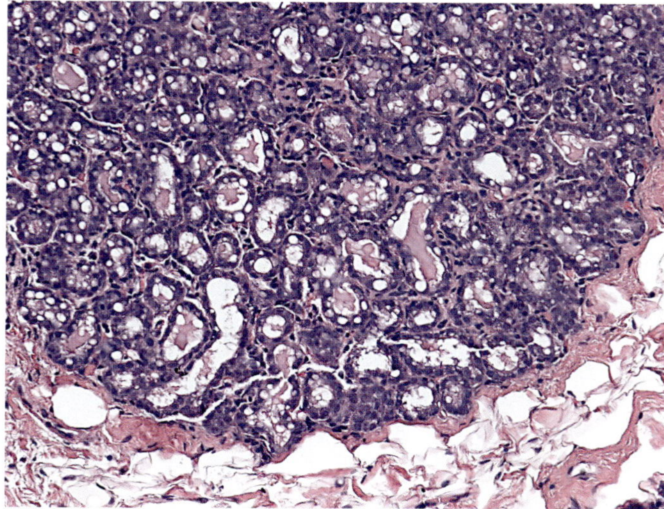

Fig. 21. Histology of lactation adenoma. This nodular lesion is composed of numerous packed small acini with dilated lumina and vacuoles within the epithelial cells. H&E. Intermediate power.

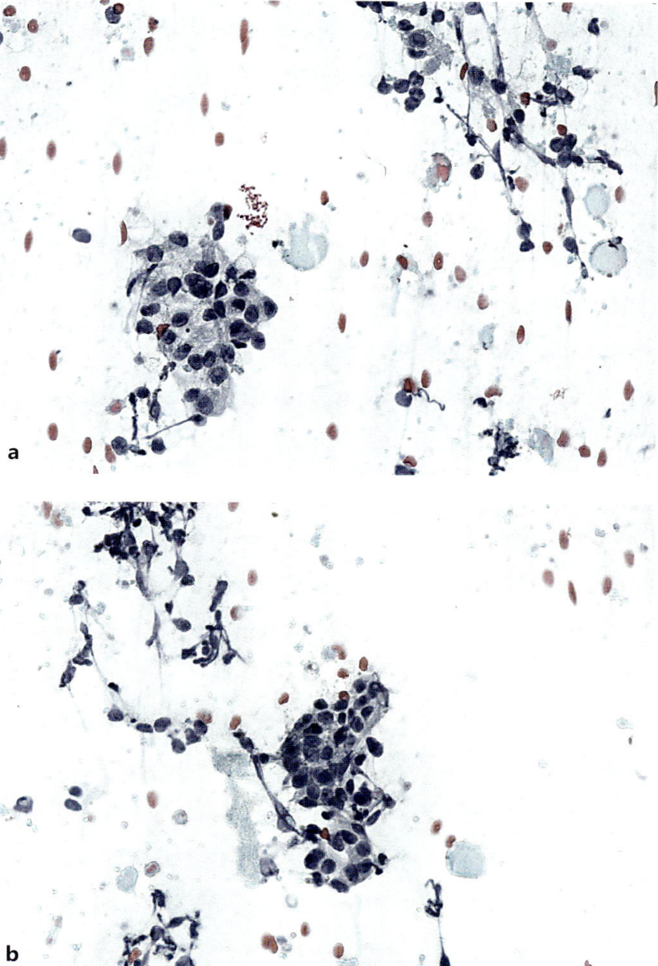

Fig. 22. Cytology of lactating adenoma. The cytological findings of this lesion might be regarded as suspicious or even malignant if the cytopathologist were not aware of the pregnancy or lactating status of the patient. Epithelial cells are arranged in small clusters with a tendency to lose cell-to-cell cohesion and may be present also isolated (**a**, **b**). Nuclei are enlarged and display prominent nucleoli, but have round or oval shape and evenly distributed chromatin. The cytoplasm is wide and pale, containing fine vacuoles (**a**). Papanicolaou. **a**, **b** High power.

Tubular Adenoma

Introduction/Epidemiology

Tubular adenoma is a rare benign tumor of the breast morphologically related to fibroadenoma. It occurs prevalently in young nonpregnant women and presents as a single, well-defined mass that may be palpable. In these patients, the mammographic and ultrasonographical findings closely resemble those of fibroadenoma, although in older patients microcalcifications have been described, and the overall findings might be interpreted as suspicious for malignancy [Soo et al., 2000].

Histological Features

Tubular adenoma appears histologically as a single, sharply demarcated, 1- to 3-cm nodule without a true capsule and consists of closely packed, small, uniform tubular structures lined by a single layer of epithelial cells and an attenuated layer of myoepithelial cells [Kumar et al., 1998]. Unlike fibroadenoma, the intralobular stroma is not prominent (Fig. 19).

Cytology

The cytological findings of tubular adenoma include the presence of many benign ductal epithelial cells arranged in 3-dimensional cohesive ball-like clusters and tubular structures with myoepithelial cells and bare bipolar nuclei in the background. Sheets of ductal cells may occasionally show a staghorn pattern like that of fibroadenoma, but the stromal component is typically scant or absent in tubular adenomas (Fig. 20).

The presence of cohesive 3-dimensional ball-like clusters and tubular structures might lead to the suspicion of a tubular carcinoma, but myoepithelial cells are typically present in the adenoma. Moreover, the tubules of tubular adenoma are small, round, and uniform, while in tubular carcinoma they tend to be irregular in size and shape, and may sometimes show mild atypia and cellular pleomorphism [Kumar et al., 1998].

Lactating Adenoma

Introduction/Epidemiology
Lactating adenoma is an uncommon benign tumor of the breast occurring in pregnant and lactating women. Its origin is controversial, probably representing the morphological changes of a preexisting tubular adenoma or fibroadenoma during pregnancy or a coalescence of hyperplastic lobules rather than a true neoplasm [Choudhuri and Singal, 2001; Heyman et al., 2014]. It is the most prevalent breast mass in young pregnant females and commonly raises issues concerning the management of breast lesions during pregnancy.

Histological Features
Histologically, lactating adenoma is a nodular mass consisting of densely packed glands composed of actively secreting cuboidal cells with intracytoplasmic vacuoles, vesicular nuclei, and evident nucleoli (Fig. 21). It might resemble a tubular adenoma or a fibroadenoma with lactation changes of the glandular component.

Cytology
FNAC of lactating adenoma shows a consistent cellular yield of epithelial cells, scattered and in small groups, with foamy to vacuolated cytoplasm and vesicular nuclei with prominent nucleoli (Fig. 22). The background shows typically abundant foamy lipoproteinaceous material [Choudhuri and Singal, 2001]. These cytological findings must be considered in the light of the pregnancy or lactating status of the woman in order not to overestimate their "atypical" appearance. On the other hand, the eventuality of a carcinoma during pregnancy must be excluded, and a histological confirmation through core needle biopsy is advisable in the presence of suspicious elements in the aspirate.

Secretory carcinoma might resemble almost completely lactation changes on cytology. An important diagnostic clue in these cases is the absence of bipolar bare nuclei in the cancer. Moreover, great importance should be given to the clinical and imaging features of the lesion [Vesoulis and Kashkari, 1998].

References

Abendroth CS, Wang HH, Ducatman BS: Comparative features of carcinoma in situ and atypical ductal hyperplasia of the breast on fine needle aspiration biopsy specimens. Am J Clin Pathol 1991;96:654–659.

Bonzanini M, Gilioli E, Brancato B, Pellegrini M, Mauri MF, Dalla Palma P: Cytologic features of 22 radial scar/complex sclerosing lesions of the breast, three of which associated with carcinoma: clinical, mammographic, and histologic correlation. Diagn Cytopathol 1997;17:353–362.

Cho EY, Oh YL: Fine-needle aspiration cytology of sclerosing adenosis of the breast. Acta Cytol 2001; 45:353–359.

Choudhury M, Singal MK: Lactating adenoma – cytomorphologic study with review of literature. Indian J Pathol Microbiol 2001;44:445–448.

Conlon N, D'Arcy C, Kaplan JB, Cordero A, Corben AD: Radial scar at image-guided needle biopsy. Is excision necessary? Am J Surg Pathol 2015;39: 779–785.

Dawson AE, Mulford DK, Sheils LA: The cytopathology of proliferative breast disease: comparison with features of ductal carcinoma in situ. Am J Clin Pathol 1995;103:438–442.

Ellis OI, Schnitt SJ, Sastre-Garau X, et al: Invasive breast carcinoma; in Tavassoli FA, Devillee P (eds): Tumours of the Breast and Female Genital Organs. Lyon, IARC Press, 2003, pp 60–62.

Elsheikh TM, Silverman JF: Follow-up surgical excision is indicated when breast core needle biopsies show atypical lobular hyperplasia or lobular carcinoma in situ: a correlative study of 33 patients with review of the literature. Am J Surg Pathol 2005;29:534–543.

Field A, Mak A: The fine needle aspiration biopsy diagnostic criteria of proliferative breast lesions: a retrospective statistical analysis of criteria for papillomas and radial scar lesions. Diagn Cytopathol 2006;35:386–397.

Finlay ME, Liston JE, Lunt LG, Young JR: Assessment of the role of ultrasound in the differentiation of radial scars and stellate carcinomas of the breast. Clin Radiol 1994;49:52–55.

Frost AR, Aksu A, Kurstin R, Sidawy MK: Can nonproliferative and proliferative breast disease without atypia be distinguished by fine-needle aspiration cytology? Cancer 1997;81:22–28.

Ganosan S, Karthik G, Joshi M, Damodaran V: Ultrasound spectrum in intraductal papillary neoplasms of breast. Br J Radiol 2006;79:843–849.

Heymann JJ, Halligan AM, Hoda SA, Facey KE, Hoda RS: Fine-needle aspiration of breast masses in pregnant and lactating women: experience with 28 cases emphasizing ThinPrep findings. Diagn Cytopathol 2014;43:188–194.

Jeffry PB, Ljung BM: Benign and malignant papillary lesions of the breast: a cytomorphological study. Am J Clin Pathol 1994;101:500–507.

Jensen RA, Page DL, Dupont WD, Rogers LW: Invasive breast cancer risk in women with sclerosing adenosis. Cancer 1989;64:1977–1983.

King TA, Scharfenberg JC, Smetherman DH, Farkas EA, Bolton JS, Fuhrman GM: A better understanding of the term radial scar. Am J Surg 2000;180: 428–432.

Kumar N, Kapila K, Verma K: Characterisation of tubular adenoma of breast – diagnostic problem in fine-needle aspirates (FNAs). Cytopathology 1998; 9:301–307.

Lakhani SR, Ellis IO, Schnitt SJ, Tan PH, van de Vijver MJ: World Health Organization classification of tumours of the breast; in World Health Organization Classification of Tumours. Lyon, IARC, 2012, vol 4.

Lim JC, Al-Masri H, Salhadar A, Xie HB, Gabram S, Wojcik EM: The significance of the diagnosis of atypia in breast fine-needle aspiration. Diagn Cytopathol 2004;31:285–288.

Loane J: Benign sclerosing lesions of the breast. Diagn Histopathol 2009;15:395–401.

Nagi CS, O'Donnell JE, Tismenetsky M, Bleiweiss IJ, Jaffer SM: Lobular neoplasia on core needle biopsy does not require excision. Cancer 2008;112: 2152–2158.

Nassar A, Conners AL, Celik B, Jenkins SM, Smith CY, Hieken TJ: Radial scar/complex sclerosing lesions: a clinicopathologic correlation study from a single institution. Ann Diagn Pathol 2015;19:24–28.

Nayar R, De Frias DV, Bourtsos EP, Sutton V, Bedrossian C: Cytological differential diagnosis of papillary pattern in breast aspirates: correlation with histology. Ann Diagn Pathol 2001;5:34–42.

Page DL, Anderson TJ: Diagnostic Histopathology of the Breast. New York, Churchill Livingstone, 1987, pp 89–103.

Purdie CA, McLean D, Stormonth E, Macaskill EJ, McCullough JB, Edwards SL, Brown DC, Jordan LB: Management of in situ lobular neoplasia detected on needle core biopsy of breast. J Clin Pathol 2010;11:987–993.

Reid-Nicholson MD, Tong G, Cangiarella JF, Moreira AL: Cytomorphologic features of papillary lesions of the male breast: a study of 11 cases. Cancer 2006;108:222–230.

Schnitt SJ, Connolly JL, Tavassoli FA, et al: Interobserver reproducibility in the diagnosis of proliferative breast lesions using standardized criteria. Am J Surg Pathol 1992;16:1133–1143.

Shin HJ, Sneige N: Is a diagnosis of infiltrating versus in situ ductal carcinoma of the breast possible in fine-needle aspiration specimens? Cancer 1998; 84:186–191.

Silverman JF, Dabbs DJ, Gilbert CF: Fine-needle aspiration cytology of adenosis tumor of the breast. With immunocytochemical and ultrastructural observations. Acta Cytol 1989;33:181–187.

Silverman J, Masood S, Ducatman BS, Wang H, Sneige N: Can FNA biopsy separate atypical hyperplasia, carcinoma in situ, and invasive carcinoma of the breast? Cytomorphologic criteria and limitations in diagnosis. Diagn Cytopathol 1993;9:713–728.

Simpson PT, Reis-Filho JS, Gale T, et al: Molecular evolution of breast cancer. J Pathol 2005;205:248–254.

Simsir A, Waisman J, Thorner K, Cangiarella J: Mammary lesions diagnosed as "papillary" by aspiration biopsy: 70 cases with follow-up. Cancer 2003; 99:156–165.

Sloane JP, Mayers MM: Carcinoma and atypical hyperplasia in radial scars and complex sclerosing lesions: importance of lesion size and patient age. Histopathology 1993;23:225–231.

Sneige N, Staerkel GA: Fine-needle aspiration cytology of ductal hyperplasia with and without atypia and ductal carcinoma in situ. Hum Pathol 1994;25: 485–492.

Soo MS, Dash N, Bentley R, Lee LH, Nathan G: Tubular adenomas of the breast: imaging findings with histologic correlation. Am J Roentgenol 2000;174: 757–761.

Sreedharanunni S, Das A, Veenu S, Srinivasan R, Singh G: Nodular sclerosing adenosis of breast: a diagnostic pitfall in fine-needle aspiration cytology. J Cytol 2013;30:49–51.

Vesoulis Z, Kashkari S: Fine needle aspiration of secretory breast carcinoma resembling lactational changes. A case report. Acta Cytol 1998;42:1032–1036.

Visscher DW, Nassar A, Degnim AC, Frost MH, Vierkant RA, Frank RD, Tarabishy Y, Radisky DC, Hartmann LC: Sclerosing adenosis and risk of breast cancer. Breast Cancer Res Treat 2014;144: 205–212.

Pinamonti M, Zanconati F: Breast Cytopathology. Assessing the Value of FNAC in the Diagnosis of Breast Lesions.
Monogr Clin Cytol. Basel, Karger, 2018, vol 24, pp 58–67 (DOI: 10.1159/000479768)

Fibroepithelial Lesions

Fibroepithelial lesions are biphasic neoplasms characterized by proliferation of both epithelial and stromal components. They are a common finding in the breast of young and adult women and are almost always benign or locally aggressive lesions. Nevertheless, their presence suggests an increased proliferative activity in the breast lobules and some of them are associated with an increased risk of breast cancer.

Fibroadenoma

Introduction/Epidemiology

Fibroadenoma is the most frequent neoplasm occurring in the breast of women of any age, being more common before the menopause with a peak of incidence between 20 and 35 years of age. The typical presentation is that of a mobile mass of rubbery to firm consistency that is usually painless or may cause tenderness in conjunction with the proliferative phase of the menstrual cycle. The mass is solitary, 0.5–3 cm in maximum diameter, but larger masses up to 20 cm have been described in younger women, and there are cases of multiple, bilateral tumors, which are more frequent in black women [Morris and Shaffer, 2007]. As many as 25% of fibroadenomas are asymptomatic and are diagnosed by mammography and ultrasound [El Wakeel and Umpleby, 2003].

Ultrasonography is the best imaging technique for the detection and characterization of fibroadenomas, while mammography has generally a limited utility, except for some sclerotic fibroadenomas with "popcorn" calcifications. The typical ultrasonographic aspect of fibroadenoma is that of a circumscribed hypoechoic homogeneous, oval-shaped mass with a long axis parallel to the skin, which may contain hyperechoic linear internal septa and be surrounded by a hyperechoic pseudocapsule resulting from the compressed adjacent breast tissue [Leconte et al., 2012].

Histological Features

Fibroadenoma is a benign, biphasic tumor consisting of a mesenchymal and an epithelial component (Fig. 1). The mesenchymal component resembles the intralobular stroma of normal breast, but is typically prominent, containing a variable population of spindle-shaped cells in a loose fibrous matrix, which may be myxoid in younger patients, becoming increasingly sclerotic and less cellular in older women. The epithelial component resembles the normal terminal ductal-lobular unit, with epithelial and myoepithelial cells. It may be hyperplastic in younger women ("juvenile" fibroadenoma) and usually involutes after the menopause, becoming atrophic and developing calcifications.

Two histologic variants are generally recognized: pericanalicular, in which ducts and acini are surrounded concentrically by connective tissue, and intracanalicular, in which the prominent stroma compresses the ducts making them appear as curvilinear slots. The distinction between these two patterns has no implications on prognosis. Fibroadenomas may also be classified as *simple* and *complex* according to the presence of associated histological features, such as cysts (>3 mm), sclerosing adenosis, duct hyperplasia with or without atypia, sometimes with papillary aspects, and apocrine changes [Carter et al., 2001]. Complex fibroadenomas are more prone to misinterpretation on cytology [Ohashi et al., 2015] and, according to some authors, carry an increased risk of developing cancer [Dupont et al., 1994].

The presence of stromal pleomorphic cells in fibroadenomas is uncommon. If it is an isolated, incidental finding in otherwise typical lesions, their presence has no clinical implications [Heneghan et al., 2008]. Nevertheless, the presence of pleomorphic stromal cells in combination with mitotic activity, stromal overgrowth, or hypercellularity raises the possibility of another lesion, usually phyllodes tumor. Occasionally, primary ductal or lobular carcinomas (in situ or invasive) may arise within a fibroadenoma [Wu et al., 2014].

Cytology

The typical aspirate from a fibroadenoma is fairly cellular, containing monolayer epithelial cell sheets, stromal tissue fragments, and many dispersed bare nuclei in an otherwise clean background [Benoit et al., 1992]. The epithelial component is represented by cohesive clusters of ductal cells with bland nuclei that frequently show a typical antler-shaped or staghorn morphology with neat borders and finger-like ends. Myoepithelial cells are easily detected above the epithelial cells. Stromal fragments are usually paucicellular and can be found isolated or attached to the epithelial layers; they may be associated with myxoid material. Bare nuclei are typically numerous in the background and have an oval or bipolar shape (Fig. 2, 3).

Beyond these classical cytological features, fibroadenomas may exhibit a variety of unusual aspects that can lead to a misinterpretation as another benign or, sometimes, malignant entity [Benoit et al., 1992; Kollur and El Haag, 2006].

These include cellular dissociation, epithelial hyperplasia, mild nuclear pleomorphism, clearly visible nucleoli, apocrine metaplasia, foamy or clear cytoplasm in epithelial cells, and multinucleated giant macrophages [Kollur and El Haag, 2006]. Moreover, the presence of hypercellularity among stromal tissue fragments can pose a difficult differential diagnosis between a "cellular" fibroadenoma and a phyllodes tumor (Fig. 3) (see below).

When the main cytological criteria (staghorn clusters of ductal epithelial cells, numerous single bare nuclei, and fragments of fibromyxoid stroma) are present, the lesion can be safely assessed as "benign lesion: fibroadenoma" (C2). The presence of suspicious elements, such as epithelial or stromal hypercellularity, nuclear pleomorphism, and cellular dissociation, should lead the cytopathologist to consider the smear as "atypical" (C3) and to discuss the case in a multidisciplinary meeting.

In the absence of suspicious elements, but lacking one or more features of the diagnostic triad, it is possible to assess the lesion as benign, even if the diagnosis of fibroadenoma is not sure.

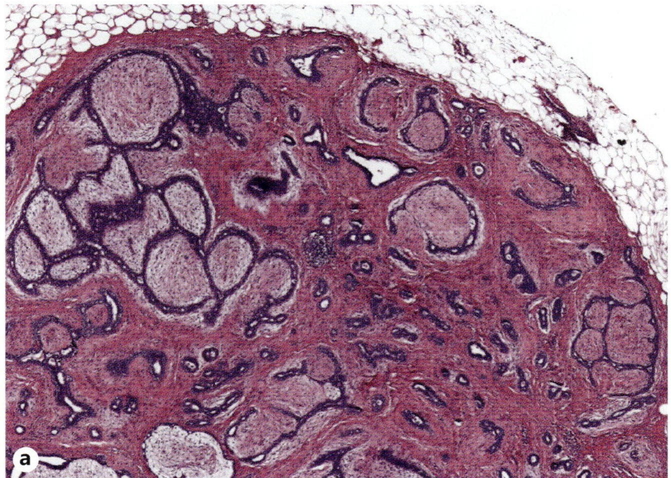

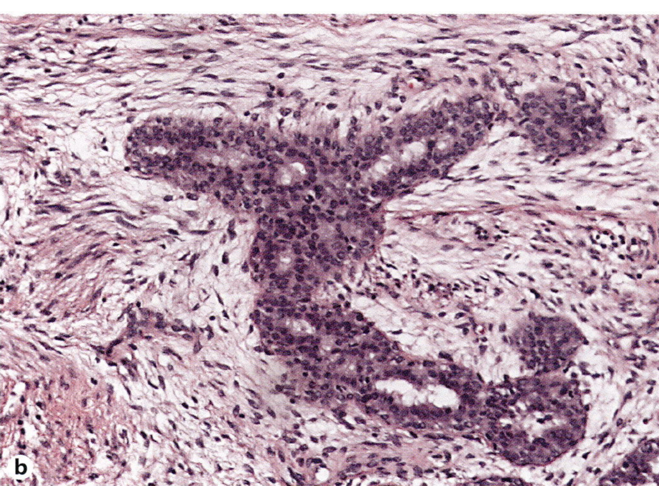

Fig. 1. Histology of fibroadenoma. Fibroadenoma is a well-circumscribed nodular mass composed of a stromal and an epithelial component. The stroma can be myxoid or fibrosclerotic and more or less cellular depending on the age and hormonal status of the woman. H&E. **a** Scanning magnification. **b** Intermediate power.

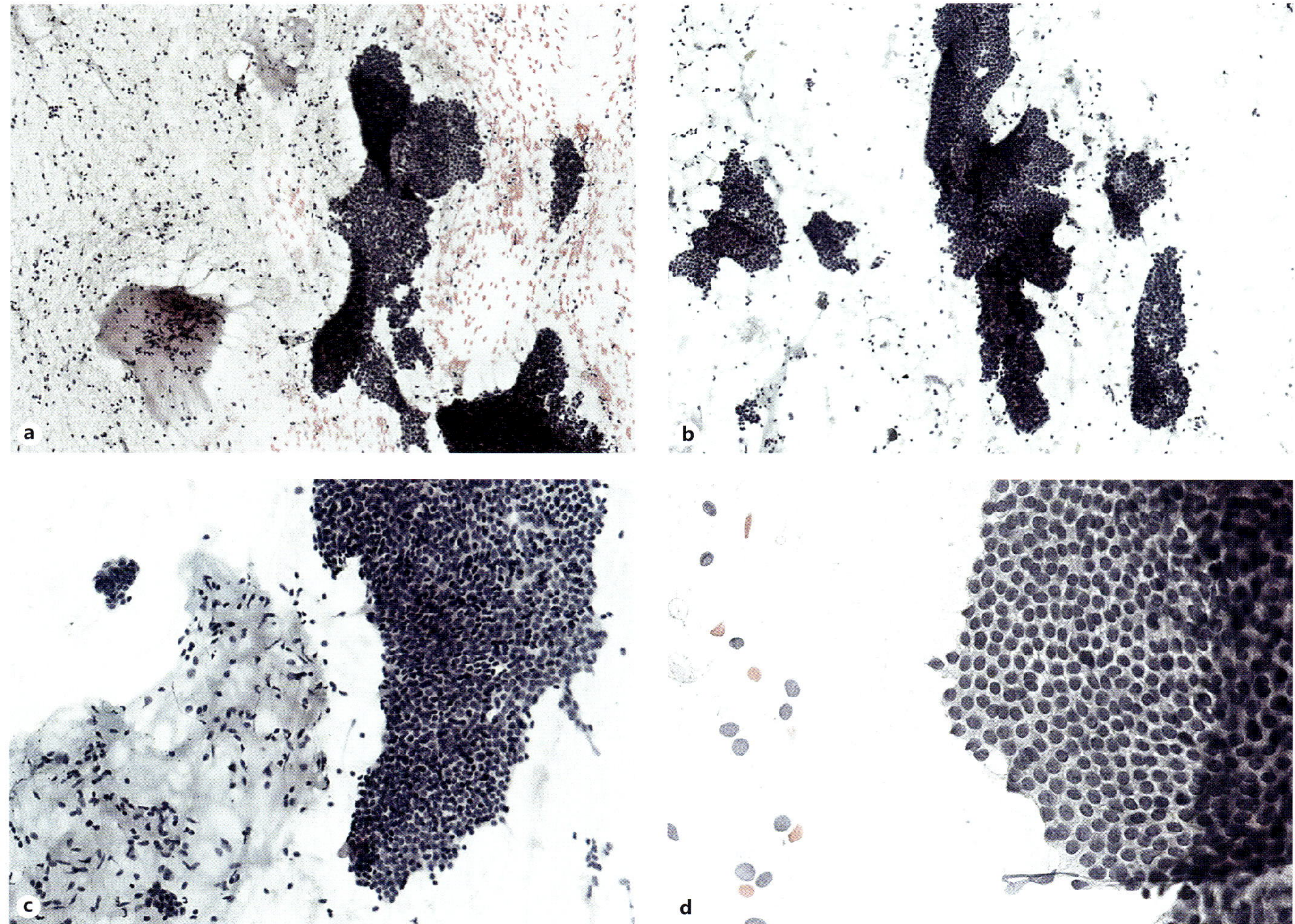

Fig. 2. Cytology of fibroadenoma. Aspirates taken from fibroadenomas are usually moderately to markedly cellular and display wide, branching monolayer epithelial sheets, stromal fragments, and many bare nuclei in the background (**a**, **b**). Epithelial layers have typically round, finger-like ends and are composed of uniform ductal cells with scattered myoepithelial cells (**c**, **d**). Stromal fragments are fibrillary or myxoid and variably cellular (**c**). Bare nuclei are typically numerous and have a distinct oval or slightly elongated shape (**d**). Papanicolaou stain. **a**, **b** Low power. **c** Intermediate power. **d** High power.

Summary

Key Cytological Features of Fibroadenoma

- Moderate to marked cellularity
- Staghorn epithelial clusters with neat borders and finger-like ends
- Myoepithelial cells
- Numerous bare bipolar nuclei
- Stromal fragments

Common Pitfalls of FNA: Fibroadenoma

- Epithelial hypercellularity
- Stromal hypercellularity
- Isolated intact epithelial cells
- Mild nuclear pleomorphism
- Myxoid matrix – similar to mucus

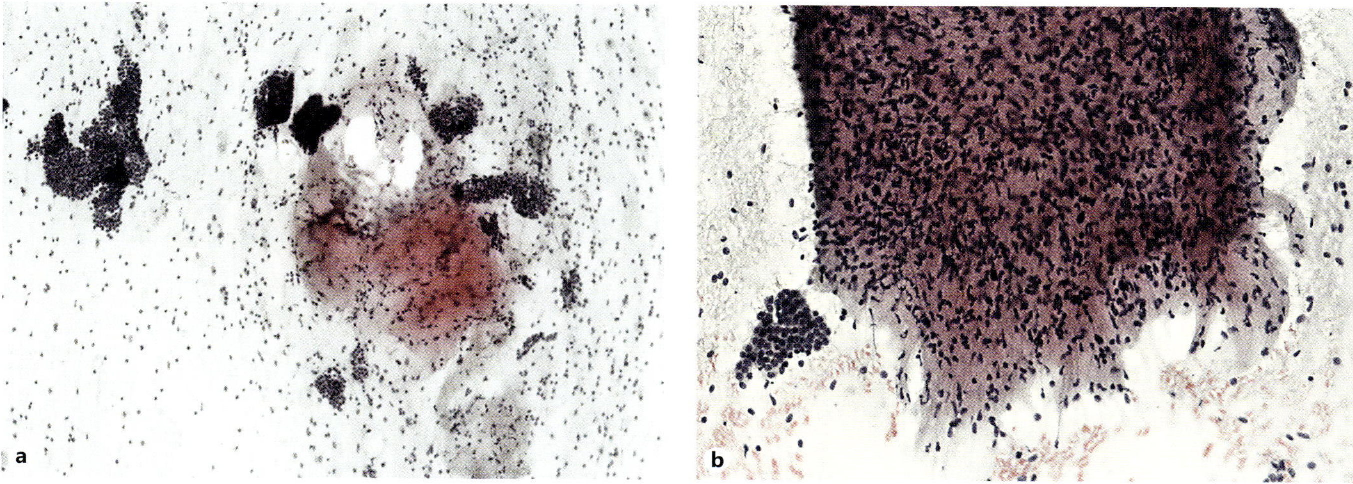

Fig. 3. Stromal features in fibroadenomas. The stromal component of fibroadenomas varies greatly from case to case and can pose some differential diagnoses. A myxoid background (**a**) might be mistaken for a mucous substance of a mucinous carcinoma, while cellular stroma (**b**) raises the suspicion of a phyllodes tumor. Papanicolaou. **a** Low power. **b** Intermediate power.

Phyllodes Tumor

Introduction/Epidemiology

Phyllodes tumor is a rare neoplasm accounting for <1% of all breast masses and 2.5% of all fibroepithelial tumors [MacDonald et al., 2006; Rosen and Oberman, 1993]. Its name derives from the Greek word phyllon, meaning leaf, for its macroscopic aspect of a leaf-shaped pattern of tumor nodules. Originally called cystosarcoma phyllodes, it is most of the times a benign or borderline neoplasm similar to fibroadenoma, with a less predictable clinical behavior and higher tendency to recur, and thus the name phyllodes tumor is preferred [Ben Hassouna et al., 2006]. Nonetheless, some cases display evident malignant features and behave like aggressive sarcomas with infiltration of local tissue, frequent recurrence, and distant metastases [Lakhani et al., 2012]. Phyllodes tumor usually presents as a well-defined palpable breast mass with a tendency to grow rapidly in few weeks. The tumor size is typically larger than that of the more common fibroadenoma (usually >4 cm), and the age of occurrence is 20 years higher (average 45 years) [MacDonald et al., 2006]. The ultrasonographic and mammographic aspects of phyllodes tumor are not significantly differen from those of fibroadenoma, and radiological imaging is generally considered unable to distinguish the two entities and the benign or malignant form of phyllodes tumor [Chao et al., 2003]. Some radiological features that are described associated more with phyllodes tumor than with fibroadenoma include the larger dimensions, absence of calcification (due to the rapid growth of the lesion), irregular or lobulated shape, and the heterogeneous parenchyma [Tan et al., 2012].

Histological Features

Like fibroadenoma, phyllodes tumor is a biphasic neoplasm with an epithelial and a mesenchymal component, with a predominance of the latter. Periductal stroma is hypercellular, with a leaf-like architectural pattern, variable nuclear atypia, and mitotic activity. These features, together with the tumor margin appearance, are the main features that allow a distinction between the benign, borderline, and malignant form [Lakhani et al., 2012]. Nevertheless, these are typically heterogeneous neoplasms, containing foci with benign, borderline, and malignant features intermingled within the same lesion. Thus, careful gross examination and histological sampling are fundamental to make the correct diagnosis [Zhang and Kleer, 2016].

Benign phyllodes tumors are characterized by mildly increased stromal cellularity compared to fibroadenomas and mild nuclear atypia (Fig. 4). Mitoses are rare, usually fewer than 5 per 10 high-power fields. These lesions may be very similar to fibroadenomas, but they have a higher rate of local recurrence. Malignant phyllodes tumor, originally called *cystosarcoma phyllodes* since its first recognition in 1938 by Müller, is characterized by stromal overgrowth with nuclear pleomorphism and more than 10 mitoses per 10 high-pow-

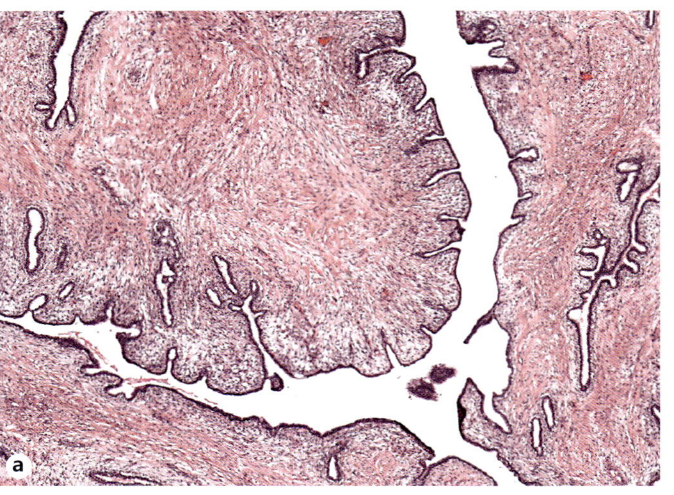

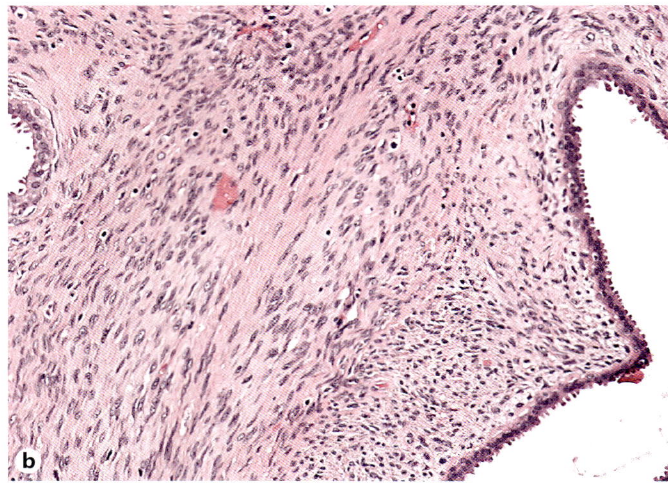

Fig. 4. Benign phyllodes tumor. This nodular lesion is composed of a prominent cellular stroma and almost normal ductal structures (**a**). At higher magnification, stromal cells show spindle morphology and are arranged in bands around the ductal structures (**b**). Mitotic activity is generally low and hard to notice. H&E. **a** Scanning magnification. **b** Intermediate power.

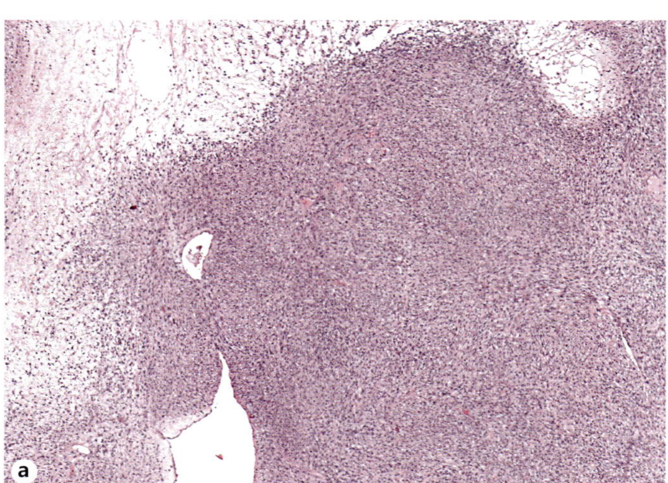

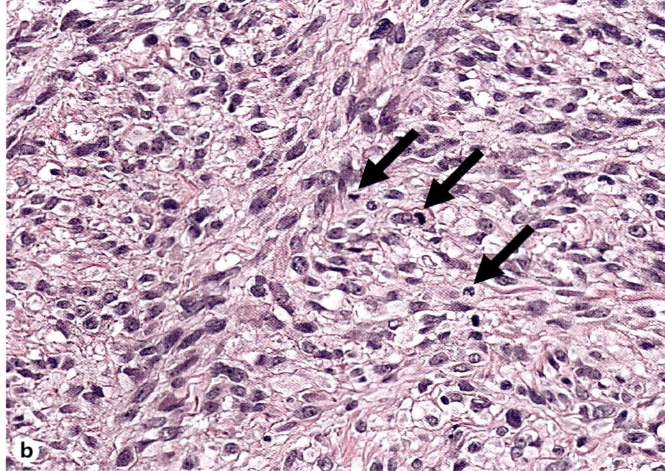

Fig. 5. Malignant phyllodes tumor. Malignant phyllodes tumors resemble high-grade sarcomas, with high stromal cellularity, necrosis (**a**), and frequent mitoses (arrows) (**b**). The epithelial component might be extremely reduced or even absent. H&E. **a** Scanning magnification. **b** High power.

er fields (Fig. 5). The presence of heterologous sarcomatous elements (liposarcoma, chondrosarcoma, and osteosarcoma) is sufficient to qualify a phyllodes tumor as malignant. Lesions displaying intermediate characteristics or not meeting all the criteria to be considered malignant are included in the *borderline* category (Fig. 6). It is characterized by a tendency to local recurrence and extreme rarity of distant metastases.

Cytology

The accuracy of fine-needle aspiration cytology in the diagnosis of phyllodes tumor is variable, with sensitivity values reported in the literature ranging from 25 to 77% [Jacklin et al., 2006; Tse et al., 2002]. Actually, the diagnosis of malignant phyllodes tumor is usually simple and does not pose much problems in the presence of marked atypia, pleomorphism, and mitotic activity among the stromal component

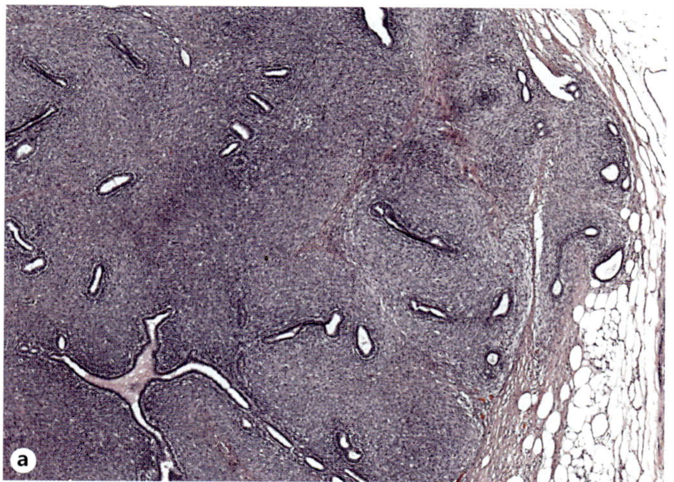

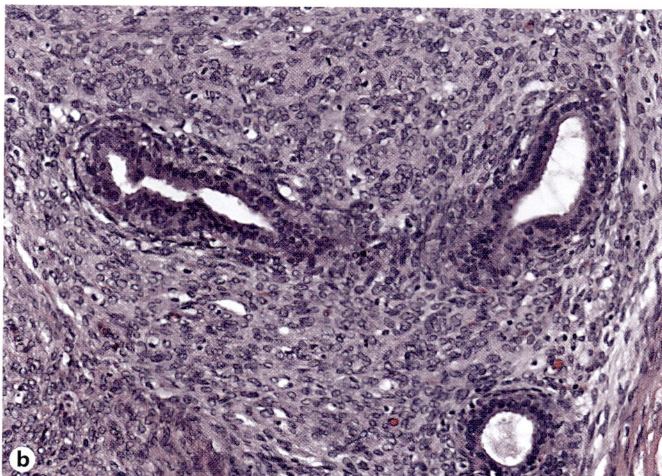

Fig. 6. Borderline phyllodes tumor. This biphasic nodule shows distinct stromal hypercellularity, still preserving some epithelial structures. Several mitotic figures are present but are not as numerous as in malignant phyllodes tumors. H&E. **a** Scanning magnification. **b** Intermediate power.

[Jayaram and Sthaneshwar, 2002]. The poor sensitivity of cytology is mainly due to the failure to recognize benign and borderline phyllodes tumors, which represent 80% of all phyllodes tumor cases.

Similar to fibroadenomas, cytological smears from benign and borderline phyllodes tumors display both epithelial and stromal elements. The epithelial component is represented by 2-dimensional layers of ductal cells with myoepithelial cells and usually does not show significant atypia. The stromal component is made up of single, dispersed, fibroblast-like spindle cells and aggregates or fragments containing spindle cells and fibrous matrix (Fig. 7). It represents the key diagnostic element to recognize phyllodes tumors and to identify their benign or malignant nature [Scolyer et al., 2001]. A bland dispersed population of cells is seen in benign phyllodes tumors, while borderline cases are characterized by the presence of atypical dispersed cells. In malignant phyllodes tumors, the epithelial component is markedly reduced or even absent, and the stromal part shows anaplastic cells and frequent mitoses. In addition, in malignant phyllodes tumors, stromal fragments tend to be large and show trabecular, anastomosing, and arborizing patterns [Jayaram and Sthaneshwar, 2002] (Fig. 8).

Aspirates suggestive for benign or borderline phyllodes tumors should be included in the "indeterminate/probably benign" category in order to stress the need for an adequate treatment: even a benign phyllodes tumor is an increasingly growing mass that needs to be excised. Moreover, the lesion is frequently inhomogeneous and foci of a malignant lesion might have not been sampled.

Aspirates with all the cytological features of a malignant phyllodes tumor (numerous pleomorphic stromal cells and frequent mitotic figures) should be included in the "malignant" category (C5) or in the "suspicious for malignancy" category (C4) in doubtful cases.

Summary

Key Cytological Features of Phyllodes Tumor

- Moderate to marked cellularity
- Benign epithelial layers (in benign and borderline tumors) admixed with a well-represented stromal component
- Stromal hypercellularity
- Elongated spindle cells

Common Pitfalls of FNA: Phyllodes Tumor

- Lack of the epithelial component
- Subtle stromal cytological atypia

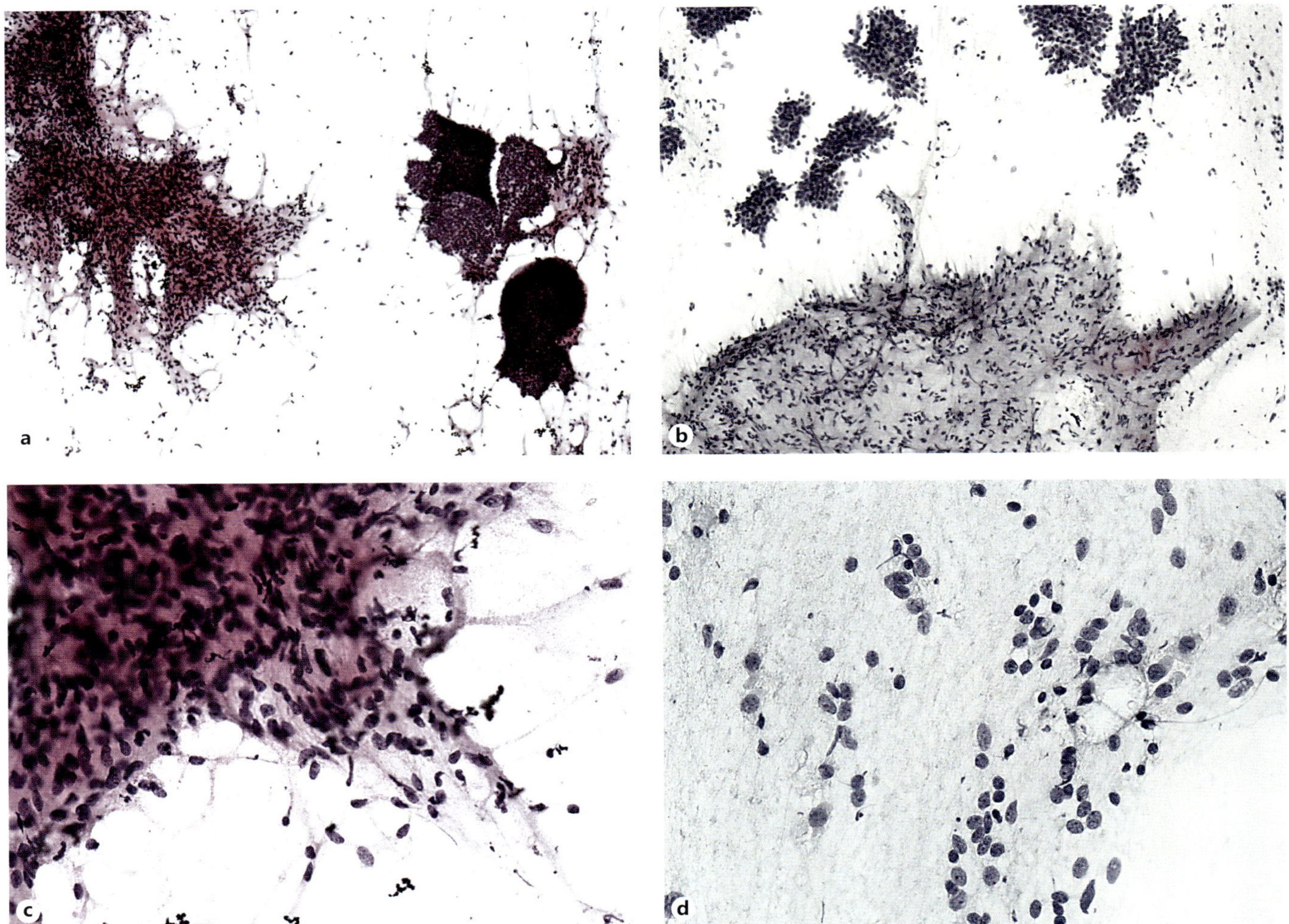

Fig. 7. Cytology of phyllodes tumor. Aspirates from benign and borderline phyllodes tumors may show variable epithelial cellularity, sometimes with the typical features of fibroadenomas (**a**) or even papillary aspects (**b**), and typically densely cellular stromal fragments. Such a stromal cellularity should be considered cautiously and assessed at least as "atypical" or "indeterminate" (C3). At higher magnification, stromal cells frequently show spindle/elongated shapes (**c**) or may be oval and plump (**d**). Papanicolaou. **a**, **b** Low power. **c**, **d** High power.

Hamartoma

Introduction/Epidemiology

Hamartoma of the breast is an uncommon benign lesion, which is said to account for approximately 4% of all benign lesions, but it is probably more frequent due to its frequent underrecognition and common misinterpretation as a fibroadenoma [Sevim et al., 2014; Williams and Williams, 1996]. It typically occurs in women older than 35 years, with a peak incidence at around 40 years of age. Its clinical presentation is that of a palpable, painless "benign-looking" mass (1–8 cm in diameter) with soft to rubbery consistency.

Mammogram is capable of identifying most breast hamartomas for the presence of the diverse tissue components, which produce a typically heterogeneous image with radiopaque and radiotransparent areas within a well-defined mass. This pecular appearance is described by radiologists with different terms, such as "bull's eye," "multi-layered," or "salami slice." The ultrasonographic aspect is that of a well-defined, oval-shaped lump with long axis parallel to the skin, showing an inhomogeneous echo pattern without posterior acoustic shadowing [Chao et al., 2007; Daya et al., 1995; Presazzi et al., 2015].

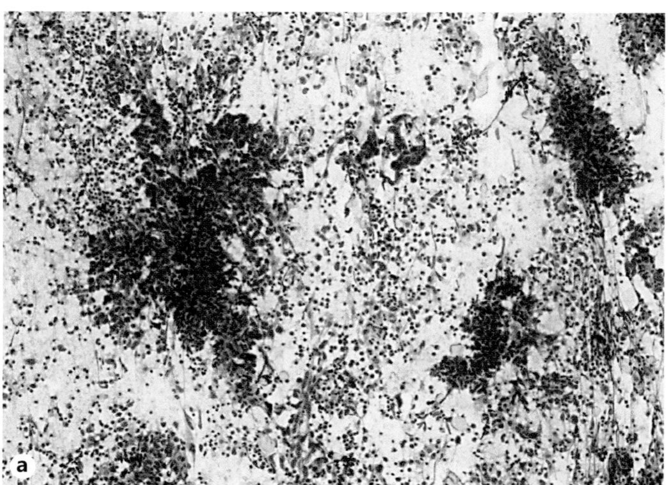

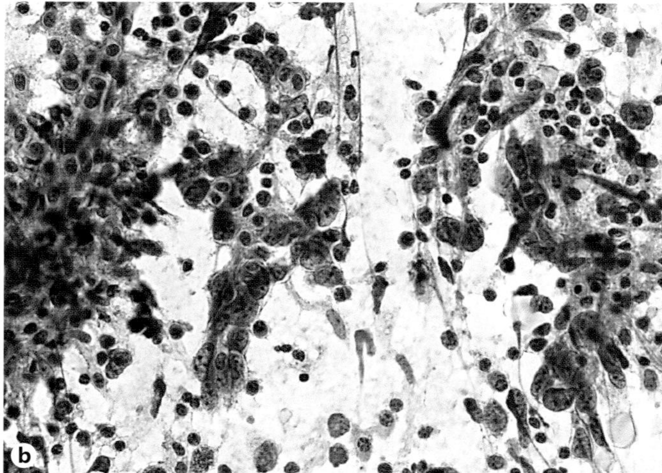

Fig. 8. Cytology of malignant phyllodes tumor. Malignant phyllodes tumor may be suspected in the presence of many severely atypical spindle-shaped elements on the smear, but this diagnosis is unreliable and not recommended, since such cells might be indistinguishable from those of other sarcomas (mainly angiosarcomas) and even some high-grade carcinomas. Still, a diagnosis of malignant neoplasm (C5) can be made with relative safety. Papanicolaou. **a** Low power. **b** High power.

Histological Features

Rather than a true neoplasm, breast hamartoma is a proliferation of normal breast tissue in a disorganized fashion, often with one predominant element [Charpin et al., 1994]. Histologically, it reproduces normal breast lobules with overgrowth of the epithelial component and various amounts of fibrotic stroma and adipose tissue interposed between glandular units. The epithelial component may contain areas of hyperplasia and cysts. The stromal component may show smooth muscle, cartilage, and brown fat tissue [Garijo et al., 1997], as well as pseudoangiomatous hyperplasia [Daya et al., 1995; Fisher et al., 1992]. It is a completely benign lesion, which does not carry an increased risk of developing cancer.

Cytology

In the daily practice, the radiological features of breast hamartomas are generally sufficient for a reliable diagnosis of benign lesion, so it is rarely subject to further examination through FNAC or biopsy. For this reason, there are few studies taking its main cytological features into consideration [Singh and Nawaz, 1998]. Aspirates from breast hamartomas are variably cellular and show an admixture of benign epithelial and mesenchymal elements. Differently from fibroadenoma, the epithelial component frequently includes intact lobular and acinar structures, and the stroma may contain fragments of fat and dense fibrous tissue with attached epithelial elements [Herbert et al., 2006]. These aspects are indistinguishable from normal breast tissue, but the finding of a well-defined mass both clinically and radiologically indicates the presence of a lesion. For this reason, the diagnosis of breast hamartoma is not possible on a breast aspirate alone and must be considered in a multidisciplinary context [Gomez-Aracil et al., 2003]. Nevertheless, the benign nature of the lesion can be safely assessed through cytology, and, in most cases, there is no need for further diagnostic procedures to grant the best management to the patient. With the exception of large masses that may cause discomfort to the patient in some cases, or lesions associated with atypical duct hyperplasia, breast hamartomas do not need any treatment.

Pseudoangiomatous Stromal Hyperplasia

Introduction/Epidemiology

Pseudoangiomatous stromal hyperplasia (PASH) is a rare benign lesion of the breast resulting from a hormone-dependent proliferation of myofibroblasts resembling a low-grade vascular lesion [Castro et al., 2002]. It may occur in premenopausal women as a palpable well-defined mass of variable size whose clinical, mammographic, and sonographic findings most often lead to the diagnosis of fibroadenoma [Hargaden et al., 2008]. PASH is a benign lesion with a variable tendency to grow causing breast asymmetry, pain, or discomfort to patients but does seem to pose an increased risk of developing breast cancer. Thus, its management is usually careful observation or conservative surgery for larger masses.

Histological Features

PASH is histologically characterized by the presence of interanastomosing angulated and slit-like spaces lined by slender spindle cells and surrounded by dense collagenous stroma. An epithelial component is typically present in the form of breast ducts entrapped in the stromal proliferation and might give this lesion an aspect similar to a fibroadenoma or a phyllodes tumor. The name „pseudoangiomatous" derives from the frequent misinterpretation as a low-grade angiosarcoma due to the presence of the ramifying slits resembling vascular structures, but these do not contain blood cells and are probably a fixation artifact induced by the retraction of the collagenous stroma. Furthermore, the lesion does not exhibit any atypia or mitotic activity. Stromal cells are typically positive for CD34, vimentin, and hormonal receptors but negative for factor VIII [Bowman et al., 2012].

Cytology

Aspirates from PASH lesions usually display a stromal and an epithelial component, sometimes in the form of "staghorn" ductal clusters, which can be very similar to those found in fibroadenomas. The presence of many elongated spindle cells or bipolar bare nuclei in the background is another element in favor of a wrong diagnosis of fibroadenoma or phyllodes tumor. Thus, FNAC findings of PASH are not specific, and a definite diagnosis cannot be made solely based on cytological findings [Lui et al., 2004].

Differential Diagnoses among Fibroepithelial Lesions

Fibroadenoma versus Benign and Borderline Phyllodes Tumor

Fibroadenoma shares many radiological, histological, and cytological aspects with benign and borderline phyllodes tumors, and the differential diagnosis between these entities can be extremely difficult. Some clinical aspects might be helpful to suspect the presence of one or the other lesion in a certain patient, but they are never conclusive. Patients with phyllodes tumor tend to be older than those with fibroadenoma, and the lesion is more frequently palpable, larger than 3 cm, and progressively growing irrespective of the menstrual cycle. When analyzing the cytological smear, the presence of high cellularity within stromal layers, stromal cytological atypia, and a low epithelial/stromal ratio are the first clues that may raise the possibility of a phyllodes tumor [Tse et al., 2002]. Some authors suggest that the presence of long, spindle nuclei in more than 30% of the dispersed stromal cells is the most reliable discriminator between the two lesions [El Hag et al., 2010; Krishnamurthy et al., 2000]. In fact, spindle cells can be seen in fibroadenomas, especially cellular ones, but do not exceed 10% of the total dispersed cell population.

As suggested by Scolyer et al. [2001], we believe that an aspirate suggestive for a fibroadenoma concomitant with hypercellular stromal fragments should be deemed as "possible phyllodes tumor" and entered in the "atypia" category in order to be histologically confirmed.

Malignant Phyllodes Tumor versus Other Sarcomas

Fibrosarcoma, malignant fibrous histiocytoma, rhabdomyosarcoma, and other rare sarcomas of the breast might be suspected in the presence of markedly atypical spindle cells in an aspirate. Nevertheless, we believe that the distinction between these entities based solely on fine-needle aspiration is unreliable and of little use in daily practice. Actually, primary sarcomas of the breast tissue are extremely rare, and the majority of mesenchymal malignancies in the breast arise as a component of a malignant phyllodes tumor [Zhang and Kleer, 2016]. Moreover, disease-free and overall survival rates of primary breast sarcoma patients are identical to those of patients with malignant phyllodes tumor, and the treatment should be the same [Wang et al., 2015].

Malignant Phyllodes Tumor versus Metaplastic Carcinoma

Metaplastic carcinoma and carcinosarcoma of the breast are other possible mimickers of malignant phyllodes tumor. Aspirates from metaplastic carcinomas may display numerous dispersed atypical epithelioid or spindle-shaped cells, as well as hypercellular clusters, mitotic figures, and a wide spectrum of heterologous sarcomatous elements. In the presence of malignant epithelial cells combined with malignant mesenchymal elements, the diagnosis of a metaplastic carcinoma or a true carcinosarcoma should be considered. Conversely, the presence of malignant stromal elements and benign-looking epithelial clusters directs more toward the diagnosis of a phyllodes tumor [Sari et al., 2015].

References

Ben Hassouna J, Damak T, Gamoudi A, Chargui R, Khomsi F, Mahjoub S, Slimene M, Ben Dhiab T, Hechiche M, Boussen H, Rahal K: Phyllodes tumors of the breast: a case series of 106 patients. Am J Surg 2006;192:141–147.

Benoit JL, Kara R, McGregor SE, Duggan MA: Fibroadenoma of the breast: diagnostic pitfalls of fine needle aspiration. Diagn Cytopathol 1992;8:643–648.

Bowman E, Oprea G, Okoli J, Gundry K, Rizzo M, Gabram-Mendola S, Manne U, Smith G, Pambuccian S, Bumpers HL: Pseudoangiomatous stromal hyperplasia (PASH) of the breast: a series of 24 patients. Breast J 2012;18:242–247.

Carter BA, Page DL, Schuyler P, Parl FF, Simpson JF, Jensen RA, Dupont WD: No elevation in long-term breast carcinoma risk for women with fibroadenomas that contain atypical hyperplasia. Cancer 2001;92:30–36.

Castro CY, Whitman GJ, Sahin AA: Pseudoangiomatous stromal hyperplasia of the breast. Am J Clin Oncol 2002;25:213–216.

Chao TC, Chao HH, Chen MF: Sonographic features of breast hamartomas. J Ultrasound Med 2007;26:447–452; quiz 453.

Chao TC, Lo YF, Chen SC, Chen MF: Phyllodes tumors of the breast. Eur Radiol 2003;13:88–93.

Charpin C, Mathoulin MP, Andrac L, et al: Reappraisal of breast hamartoma. A morphological study of 41 cases. Path Res Pract 1994;190:362–371.

Daya D, Trus T, D'Souza TJ, Minuk T, Yemen B: Hamartoma of the breast, an under-recognized breast lesion: a clinicopathologic and radiographic study of 25 cases. Am J Clin Pathol 1995;103:685–689.

Dupont WD, Page DL, Parl FF, Vnencak-Jones CL, Plummer WD Jr, Rados MS, Schuyler PA: Long-term risk of breast cancer in women with fibroadenoma. N Engl J Med 1994;331:10–15.

El Hag IA, Aodah A, Kollur SM, Attallah A, Mohamed AAE, Al-Hussaini H: Cytological clues in the distinction between phyllodes tumor and fibroadenoma. Cancer Cytopathol 2010;118:33–40.

El-Wakeel H, Umpleby HC: Systematic review of fibroadenoma as a risk factor for breast cancer. Breast 2003;12:302–307.

Fisher CJ, Hanby AM, Robinson L, Millis RR: Mammary hamartoma: a review of 35 cases. Histopathology 1992;20:99–106.

Garijo MF, Torio B, Val-Bernal F: Mammary hamartoma with brown adipose tissue. Gen Diagn Pathol 1997;143:243–246.

Gomez-Aracil V, Mayayo E, Azua J, Mayayo R, Azua-Romeo J, Arraiza A: Fine needle aspiration cytology of mammary hamartoma: a review of nine cases with histological correlation. Cytopathology 2003;14:195–200.

Hargaden GC, Yeh ED, Georgian-Smith D, et al: Analysis of the mammographic and sonographic features of pseudoangiomatous stromal hyperplasia. Am J Roentgenol 2008;191:359–363.

Heneghan HM, Martin ST, Casey M, Tobbia I, Benani F, Barry KM: A diagnostic dilemma in breast pathology – benign fibroadenoma with multinucleated stromal giant cells. Diagn Pathol 2008;3:1–7.

Herbert M, Mendlovic S, Liokumovich P, Segal M, Zahavi S, Rath-Wolfson L, Sandbank J: Can hamartoma of the breast be distinguished from fibroadenoma using fine-needle aspiration cytology? Diagn Cytopathol 2006;34:326–329.

Jacklin RK, Ridgway PF, Ziprin P, Healy V, Hadjiminas D, Darzi A: Optimising preoperative diagnosis in phyllodes tumour of the breast. J Clin Pathol 2006;59:454–459.

Jayaram G, Sthaneshwar P: Fine needle aspiration cytology of phyllodes tumour. Diagn Cytopathol 2002;26:222–227.

Kollur SM, El Haag IA: FNA of breast fibroadenoma: observer variability and review of cytomorphology with cytohistological correlation. Cytopathology 2006;17:239–244.

Krishnamurthy S, Ashfaq R, Shin HJ, Sneige N: Distinction of phyllodes tumour from fibroadenoma: a reappraisal of an old problem. Cancer 2000;90:342–349.

Lakhani SR, Ellis IO, Schnitt SJ, Tan PH, van de Vijver MJ: World Health Organization classification of tumours of the breast; in World Health Organization Classification of Tumours. Lyon, IARC, 2012, vol 4.

Leconte I, Abraham C, Galant C, Sy M, Berlière M, Fellah L: Fibroadenoma: can fine needle aspiration biopsy avoid short term follow-up? Diagn Interv Imaging 2012;93:750–756.

Lui PC, Law BK, Chu WC, Pang LM, Tse GM: Fine-needle aspiration cytology of pseudo-angiomatous stromal hyperplasia of the breast. Diagn Cytopathol 2004;30:353–355.

Macdonald OK, Lee CM, Tward JD, Chappel CD, Gaffney DK: Malignant phyllodes tumor of the female breast: association of primary therapy with cause-specific survival from the Surveillance, Epidemiology, and End Results (SEER) program. Cancer 2006;107:2127–2133.

Morris A, Shaffer K: Recurrent bilateral giant fibroadenomas of the breasts. Radiol Case Rep 2007;2:96.

Ohashi R, Matsubara M, Watarai Y, Yanagihara K, Yamashita K, Tsuchiya SI, Takei H, Naito Z: Cytological features of complex type fibroadenoma in comparison with non-complex type fibroadenoma. Breast Cancer 2016;23:724–731.

Presazzi A, Di Giulio G, Calliada F: Breast hamartoma: ultrasound, elastosonographic, and mammographic features. Mini pictorial essay. J Ultrasound 2015;18:373–377.

Rosen PP, Oberman HA: Tumors of the Mammary Gland. Washington, Armed Forces Institute of Pathology, 1993.

Sari A, Çakalagaoğlu F, Altinboğa AA, Kucukzeybek BB, Calli A, Atahan MK: Cytopathological features of matrix-producing carcinoma of the breast. J Cytol 2015;32:33–35.

Scolyer RA, McKenzie PR, Achmed D, Leea CS: Can phyllodes tumours of the breast be distinguished from fibroadenomas using fine needle aspiration cytology? Pathology 2001;33:437–443.

Sevim Y, Kocaay AF, Eker T, Celasin H, Karabork A, Erden E, Genc V: Breast hamartoma: a clinicopathological analysis of 27 cases and a literature review. Clinics (Sao Paulo) 2014;69:515–523.

Singh M, Nawaz S: Fine needle aspiration of breast hamartoma. Acta Cytol 1998;42:437–438.

Tan H, Zhang S, Liu H, Peng W, Li R, Gu Y, Wang X, Mao J, Shen X: Imaging findings in phyllodes tumors of the breast. Eur J Radiol 2012;81:e62–e69.

Tse GM, Ma TK, Pang LM, Cheung H: Fine needle aspiration cytologic features of mammary phyllodes tumors. Acta Cytol 2002;46:855–863.

Wang F, Jia Y, Tong Z: Comparison of the clinical and prognostic features of primary breast sarcomas and malignant phyllodes tumor. Jpn J Clin Oncol 2015;45:146–152.

Williams NP, Williams E: Mammary hamartoma: an under-recognised breast lesion. West Indian Med J 1996;45:67–69.

Wu YT, Chen ST, Chen CJ, Kuo YL, Tseng LM, Chen DR, Kuo SJ, Lai HW: Breast cancer arising within fibroadenoma: collective analysis of case reports in the literature and hints on treatment policy. World J Surg Oncol 2014;12:335.

Zhang Y, Kleer CG: Phyllodes tumor of the breast: histopathologic features, differential diagnosis, and molecular/genetic updates. Arch Pathol Lab Med 2016;140:665–671.

Pinamonti M, Zanconati F: Breast Cytopathology. Assessing the Value of FNAC in the Diagnosis of Breast Lesions.
Monogr Clin Cytol. Basel, Karger, 2018, vol 24, pp 68–93 (DOI: 10.1159/000479769)

Invasive Carcinoma

Invasive breast cancer is the most common carcinoma in women, accounting for 23% of all cancers worldwide [Ferlay et al., 2008]. Its incidence increases with age and varies markedly in different geographical areas due to different lifestyles and genetic factors. Australia, Europe, and North America are the regions with the highest incidence, where 6% of women develop invasive breast cancer before 75 years of age. Although it is a widespread disease, patient prognosis is usually good when it is discovered at an early stage. Nevertheless, some subtypes of breast carcinoma behave in a very aggressive way regardless of their size. FNAC is able to identify most breast cancers with high accuracy, and there are also grounds for its routine use in the molecular and genetic characterization of tumor cells without resorting to more invasive techniques [see Chapter 11, this vol., pp. 108–111].

This chapter illustrates the main forms of breast cancer, setting the basis for the diagnosis of malignancy on FNAC and providing some hints to direct the cytological interpretation towards one or the other specific type of carcinoma.

Invasive Ductal Carcinoma and High-Grade Ductal Carcinoma in situ

Introduction/Epidemiology

Invasive ductal carcinoma of no special type (NST) is the prototype of breast cancer and accounts for approximately 40–75% of all invasive carcinomas in published series, with a wide range of variation based mostly on the strictness of the criteria used for inclusion in the other "special" types [Lakhani et al., 2012]. It is actually a heterogeneous category gathering all the invasive epithelial neoplasms lacking the characteristics to be diagnosed as a specific histological type, such as tubular or lobular. The epidemiology of ductal carcinoma NST reflects the general distribution of the breast cancer group as a whole, being rare in women younger than 40 years without a familiar or genetic predisposition and increasing in incidence with advancing age. Invasive ductal carcinomas are part of a multifocal lesion in approximately 20% of cases.

Invasive ductal carcinoma can be seen on mammography as an opacity with irregular, stellate, or nodal configuration and moderately or ill-defined contours, commonly showing calcifications. Ultrasound typically shows a hypoechoic mass with irregular shape, spiculated, indistinct, or microlobulated margins and posterior acoustic shadowing or enhancement (Fig. 1) [Blaichman et al., 2012]. Lesions larger than 2 cm, or even smaller if localized superficially or in a small breast, are often palpable and clinically detected as hard nodules. Advanced tumors may drastically alter the breast consistency and appearance, cause skin and nipple retraction or ulceration, and eventually result in the dramatic clinical presentation of inflammatory carcinoma, resembling acute mastitis.

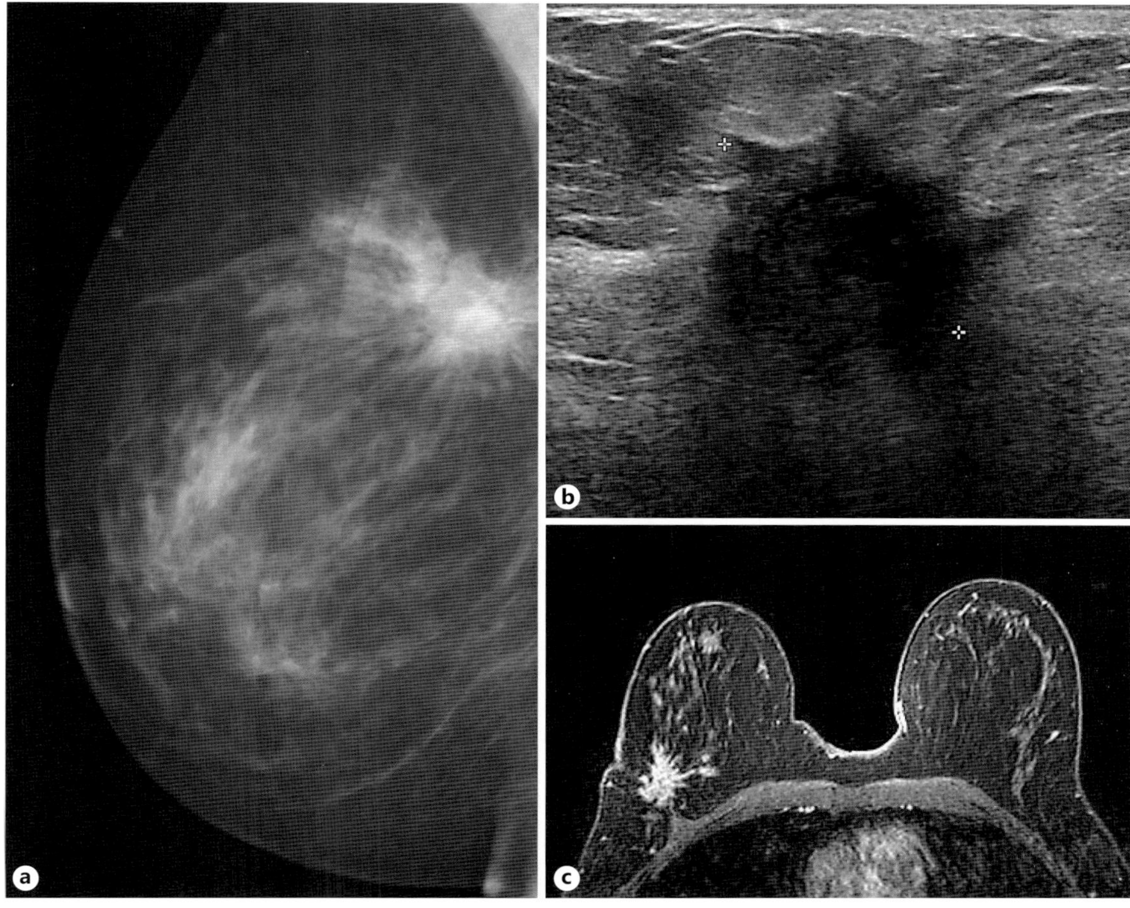

Fig. 1. Imaging of invasive ductal carcinoma. This lesion is located in the upper-outer quadrant of the right breast and is visible as a stellate opacity on mammography (**a**). Ultrasound shows a hypoechoic lesion with irregular borders and posterior acoustic shadowing (**b**). The lesion is highly suspicious also on magnetic resonance imaging (**c**).

High-grade ductal carcinoma in situ (DCIS) is a noninvasive neoplastic proliferation of ductal cells characterized by marked cytological atypia and frequently by the presence of necrosis and calcifications. Pure DCIS was considered a rare entity in the past, but, recently, its incidence has increased from 4 to nearly 25% of all breast malignancies, since the more widespread introduction of mammographic screening [Patnick, 2010]. Indeed, DCIS seldom gives rise to a palpable mass and does not generate a desmoplastic reaction, so it can only be detected by mammography in the presence of coarse, pleomorphic, and branched microcalcifications. The lack of both a palpable mass and an ultrasound-detectable nodule renders a subsequent FNAC unlikely and makes other diagnostic techniques more suitable, such as vacuum-assisted core needle biopsy under stereotaxic guidance [Jackman and Rodriguez-Soto, 2006].

Histological Features

Invasive ductal carcinoma NST may show a variety of morphological aspects encompassing different degrees of cell differentiation and architectural patterns. The tumor cells may be arranged in tubular structures, cords, clusters, or trabeculae, or occasionally infiltrate the surrounding stroma in single-cell-thick Indian files (Fig. 2). Cells may have abundant eosinophilic or scant cytoplasm, and nuclei can be regular and uniform or highly pleomorphic with prominent, multiple nucleoli. Mitotic activity may be virtually absent or extensive. The modified Bloom-Richardson-Elston grading system (also called the Nottingham system) can be used to classify invasive ductal carcinomas into 3 grades of differentiation that correlate with their aggressiveness [Elston and Ellis, 1991]. It is based on architectural criteria (rate of tubule formation/resemblance to normal breast

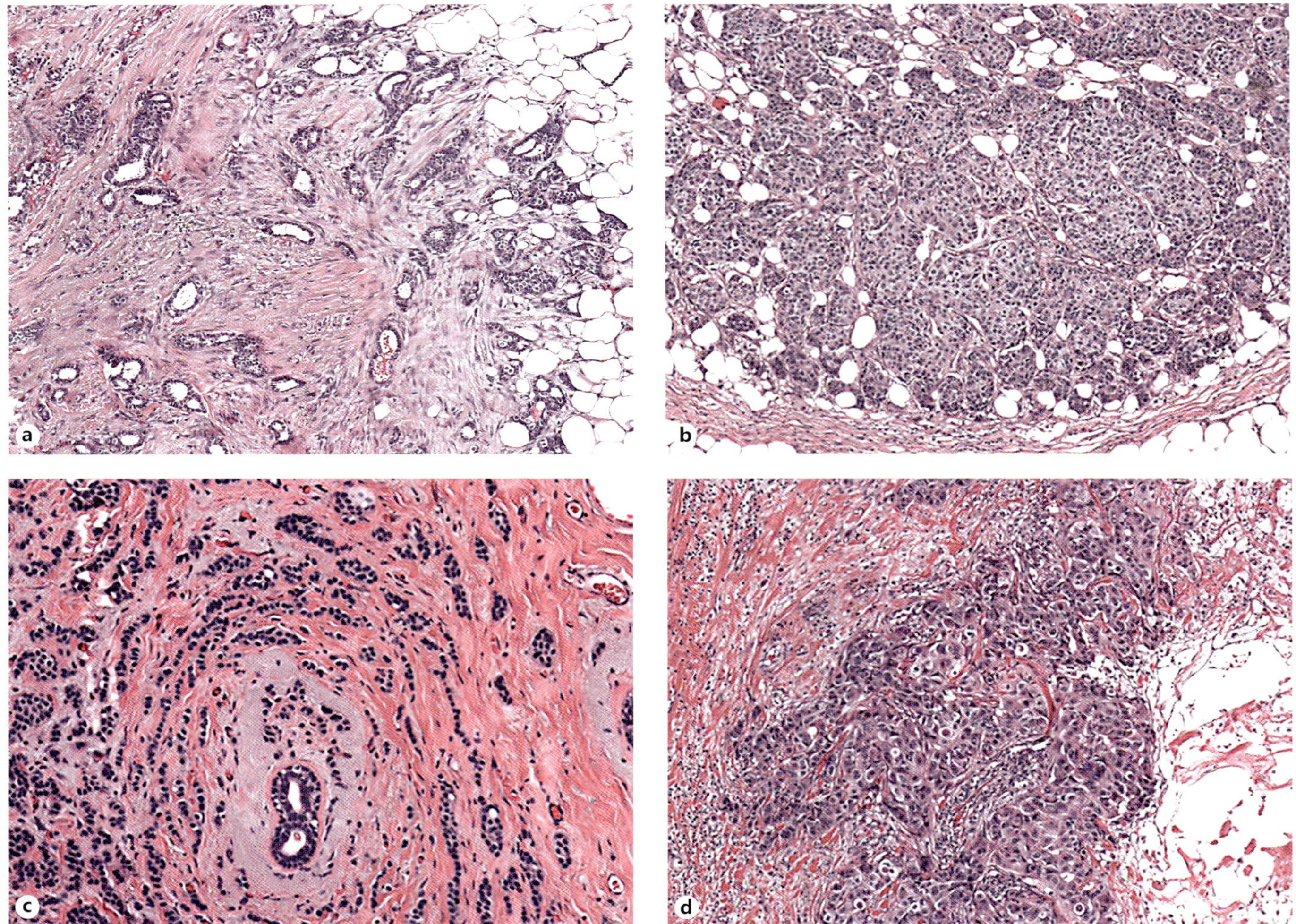

Fig. 2. Histological aspects of invasive ductal carcinoma. Well-differentiated ductal carcinomas are composed predominantly of tubular and acinar structures lined by a single layer of cuboidal cells lacking the myoepithelial component, immersed in a desmoplastic stroma (**a**). Moderately differentiated carcinomas may have a solid/trabecular architecture (**b**) or grow in single cells that infiltrate the stroma and surround normal ducts creating a sort of "target" image (**c**). Poorly differentiated cancers have solid architecture and show marked cellular atypia (**d**). H&E. Low power.

gland), combined with cytological features (nuclear atypia), and the mitotic index. Intratumor necrosis, desmoplastic reaction, and chronic inflammation are variably present in invasive ductal carcinomas and have a lesser role in defining its prognosis.

Immunohistochemistry is necessary to determine the prognosis and response of invasive ductal carcinomas NST to treatment. Hormonal receptors (estrogen and progesterone) are positive in 70–80% of cases, while human epithelial growth factor receptor 2 (HER2) is overexpressed in approximately 15% of all invasive ductal carcinomas NST [Lakhani et al., 2012].

High-grade DCIS is a proliferation of markedly atypical neoplastic cells lining the walls of breast milk ducts that may have a *solid*, *cribriform*, *papillary*, or *micropapillary* configuration. The term *comedo* is used for high-grade DCIS showing abundant necrotic debris in duct lumina (somewhat like skin blackheads or *comedones*), which may calcify (Fig. 3). Unlike the low-grade form, high-grade DCIS shows pleomorphic and poorly polarized nuclei with irregular contours, coarse, and clumped chromatin, and prominent nucleoli. In a considerable percentage of cases, high-grade DCIS is associated with an invasive component [Lakhani et al., 2012].

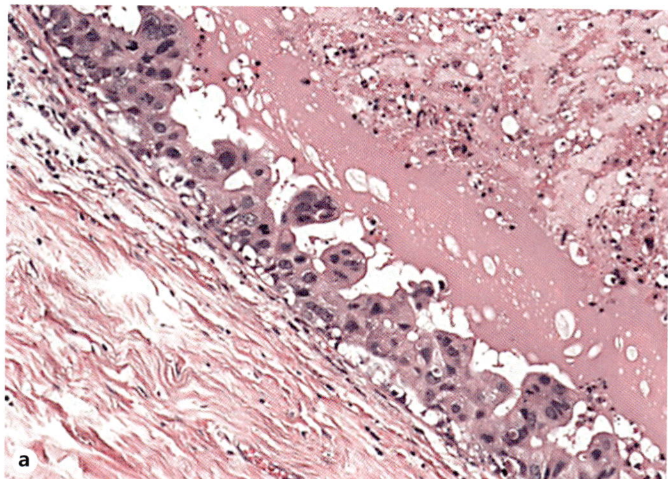

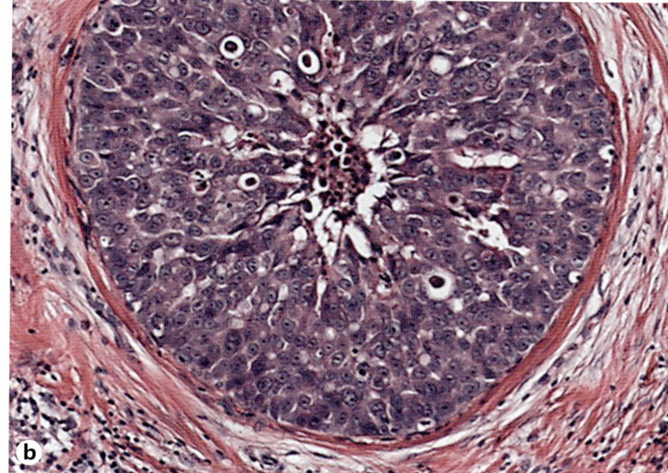

Fig. 3. High-grade ductal carcinoma in situ (DCIS). The lesion is composed of markedly atypical cells confined to the basal membrane and may show different architectural patterns: small projections of cancer cells without fibrovascular cores characterize the micropapillary variant of DCIS (**a**), while *comedo* DCIS is made up of solid nests with necrotic material in the center (**b**). H&E. Intermediate power.

Cytology

The cellular material aspirated from invasive ductal carcinoma NST is typically polymorphic, showing cells with differently shaped nuclei, which can vary in size from 1.5 to 2 times the diameter of a red blood cell to even 5 times that size. Neoplastic elements are arranged in loosely cohesive monolayers or in 3-dimensional aggregates with irregular distribution and overlapping of nuclei (Fig. 4). Occasional tubular or acinar structures may be present, especially in well- or moderately differentiated cancers (Fig. 5). Myoepithelial cells are lost in the invasive component, but they might be preserved in DCIS. In such cases, great attention must be paid to nuclear abnormalities and cellular crowding. The cells within the neoplastic clusters show loss of polarity and nuclear molding; the nuclei have irregular contours and uneven distribution of the chromatin and can be eccentrically placed, giving the cells a plasmacytoid appearance. The smears are usually highly cellular and may contain a necrotic background.

Distinguishing invasive carcinoma from high-grade DCIS in cytology is challenging and most of the times not possible in daily practice. In the setting of mammographic calcifications without a tumor detectable through ultrasound, the association of necrotic background, 3-dimensional solid aggregates of markedly atypical cells, and absence of tubular aggregates are very suggestive of the presence of DCIS [Bonzanini et al., 2001]. Also, in the presence of a palpable mass or a clearly detectable hypoechoic lesion on ultrasound, the same cytological findings should remind the cytopathologist of an invasive neoplasm.

It is possible to assess grading on cytological smears, and it correlates well with the grading made on histological samples [Robinson et al., 1994]. Neoplastic cells from well-differentiated invasive ductal carcinomas are usually smaller and less pleomorphic, resembling benign ductal cells. They display mild nuclear atypia and are arranged in cohesive monolayers or in 3-dimensional clusters with tubular or finger-like appearance. Scant isolated elements might be present, while bare nuclei are rare. Nuclear chromatin is evenly distributed, and nucleoli are small or inconspicuous. The presence of scattered less-differentiated elements may be useful for the correct diagnosis, as well as the "pointed" shape of the cell layers (Fig. 6).

Poorly differentiated invasive carcinoma is easier to recognize as malignant. Cytological abnormalities are obvious, with very large cells, polymorphic naked nuclei, and unevenly distributed chromatin, often with macronucleoli (Fig. 7). In such cases, a differential diagnosis should be made with high-grade lymphomas, metastatic melanomas, or sarcomas [see Chapter 9, this vol., pp. 94–99].

Since ductal carcinoma is a heterogeneous neoplasm, many other cytological aspects are possible. Cellular clusters may show papillary features or form cribriform gland-like structures; cancer cells may be mainly isolated or display in a linear arrangement simulating that of lobular carcinoma. Signet-ring cells may occasionally be seen.

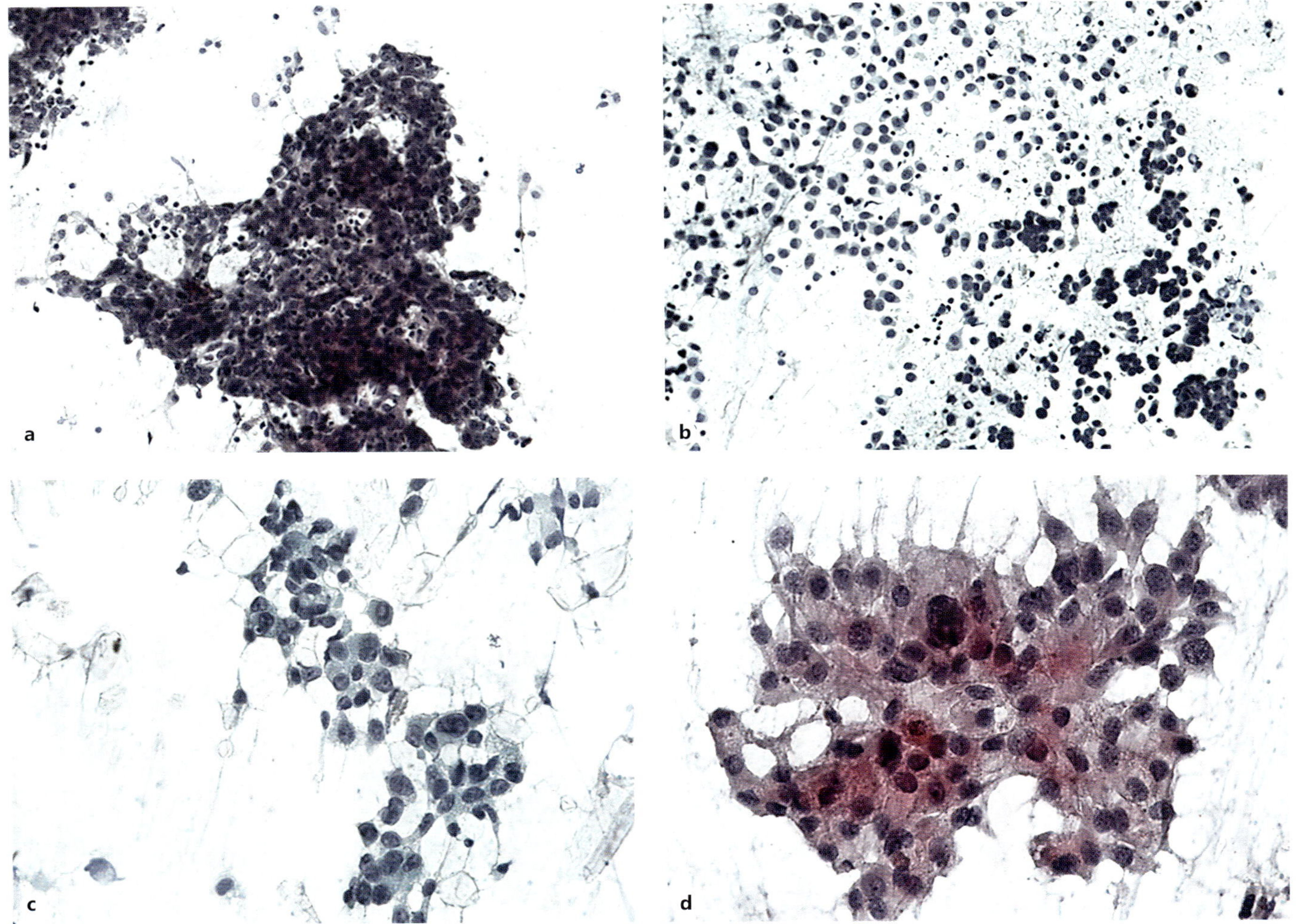

Fig. 4. Cytology of invasive ductal carcinoma of no special type. Ductal carcinoma may be suspected already at low-power magnification for the presence of irregular, 3-dimensional cell clusters (**a**) or increased cell dispersion in the smear (**b**). At higher magnification, cancer cells show a wide spectrum of nuclear abnormalities: different size and shape of nuclei, irregular chromatin distribution, and prominent nucleoli (**c**, **d**). Papanicolaou. **a**, **b** Intermediate power. **c**, **d** High power.

Summary

Key Cytological Features of Ductal Carcinoma

- High Cellularity
- Cells with different size and shape, usually large, with high nuclear/cytoplasmic ratio
- Irregular, crowded cellular clusters without myoepithelial cells
- Isolated neoplastic cells and loosely cohesive cell layers
- Hyperchromatic nuclei with irregular contours and uneven chromatin distribution

Common Pitfalls of FNA: Ductal Carcinoma

- Mild cellular atypia in low-grade cancers
- Myoepithelial cells in DCIS
- Contemporary presence of benign ductal cell layers
- Isolated cells and linear arrangement may be misleading (lobular carcinoma?)

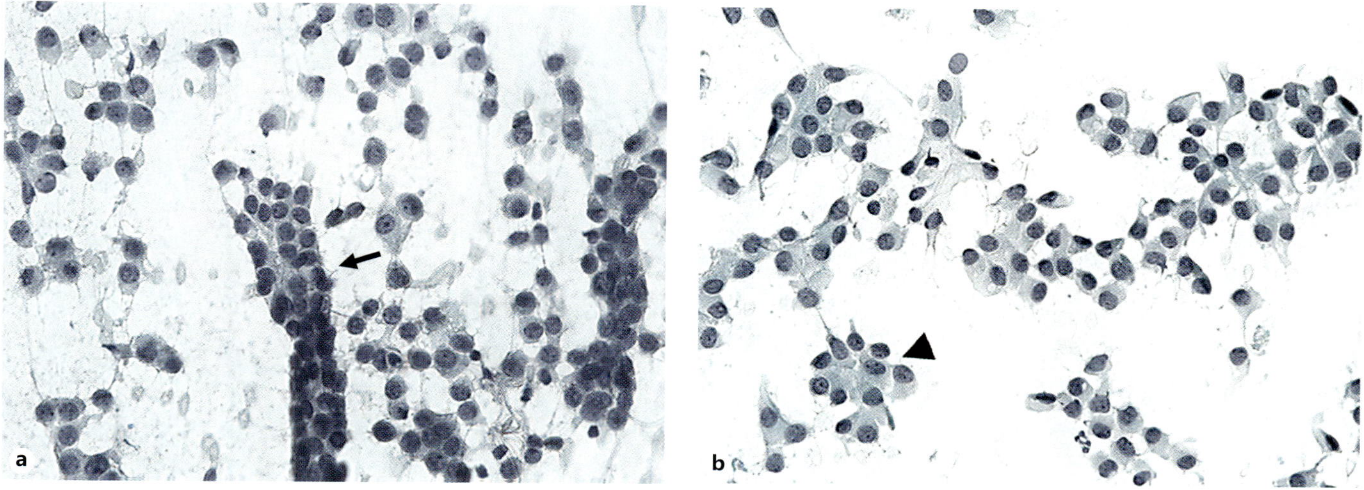

Fig. 5. Invasive ductal carcinoma of no special type. Cells of well- and moderately differentiated ductal carcinomas usually arrange in loosely cohesive small groups, tubules (arrow) (**a**), or even small, acinar-like structures (arrowhead) (**b**). Papanicolaou. High power.

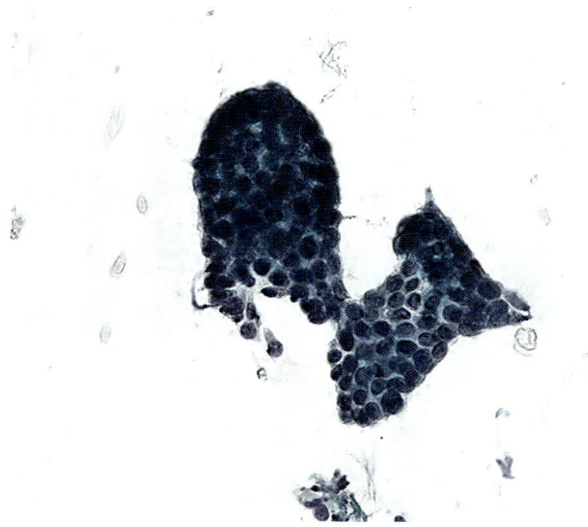

Fig. 6. Well-differentiated ductal carcinoma. It is difficult to assess this lesion as clearly malignant due to the good cohesion and monomorphism of cancer cells. Attention must be paid to the absence of myoepithelial cells and pointed edges of cellular clusters. Papanicolaou. High power.

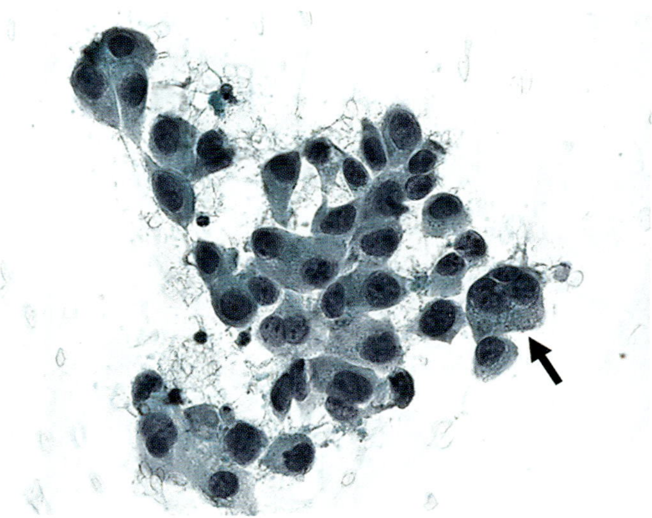

Fig. 7. Poorly differentiated ductal carcinoma. Cancer cells lack cohesion and show severe anisonucleosis and multiple, prominent nucleoli. Some cells also show binucleation (arrow). Note that the presence of abundant cytoplasm, resulting in a normal nuclear/cytoplasmic ratio, is not a reliable sign of benignity. Papanicolaou. High power.

Invasive Lobular Carcinoma

Introduction/Epidemiology

Invasive lobular carcinoma is the most common special histotype of breast carcinoma and accounts for 10–15% of all breast malignancies [Fu et al., 1998]. It usually appears in women aged 45–55 years as an ill-defined palpable mass in any of the breast quadrants and can be seen at mammography as a spiculated opacity or an architectural distortion of breast tissue [Helvie et al., 1993]. Calcifications are infrequent. Lobular carcinomas are more frequently multifocal and bilateral than ductal carcinomas, and magnetic resonance imaging can be helpful to identify multiple neoplastic foci [Hofmeyer et al., 2012].

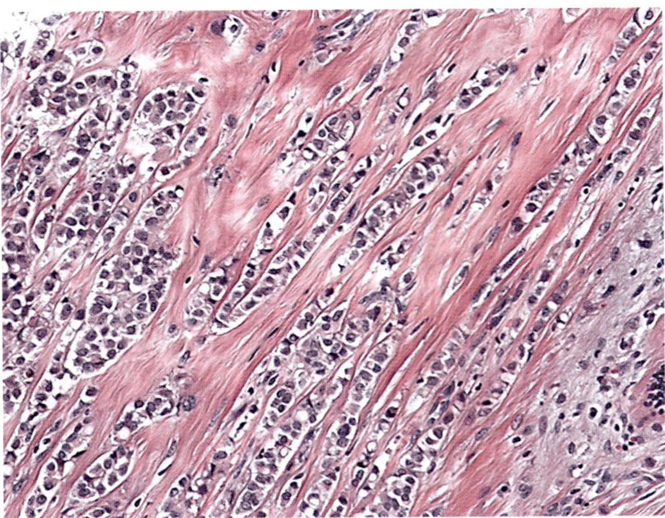

Fig. 8. Histology of invasive lobular carcinoma. Neoplastic cells infiltrate the fibrous stroma in cords or single-cell-thick Indian files. The architecture is that of a grade 3 ductal carcinoma (no duct formation), but nuclei are rather small and monomorphic, and mitotic activity is inconspicuous. H&E. Intermediate power.

Histological Features

Invasive lobular carcinoma is composed of a monotonous population of small- to medium-sized round cells with a thin rim of cytoplasm infiltrating the stroma as Indian files, small nests, and single cells lacking cellular cohesion (Fig. 8). It is typical for these linear cords of neoplastic cells to grow in a concentric pattern around normal ducts designing a sort of "target." Necrosis is usually absent, and mitotic figures are rare [Toikkanen et al., 1997].

The rare *pleomorphic* variant of lobular carcinoma has a greater degree of cellular atypia and pleomorphism and a higher mitotic activity. It may show apocrine or histiocytoid differentiation and may be composed of signet-ring cells [Eusebi et al., 1992; Walford and ten Velden, 1989].

Cancer cells from lobular carcinoma do not express E-cadherin on their membrane and are thus recognizable through immunohistochemistry [Pai et al., 2013]. Lobular neoplasms are typically moderately differentiated (grade 2), express hormonal receptors, and are HER2 negative (0) or weakly positive (1+), except for the pleomorphic variant, which is more frequently progesterone negative and HER2 positive [Arpino et al., 2004].

Cytology

Invasive lobular carcinoma is often difficult to recognize in cytological preparations due to the small size and monomorphism of cancer cells, which may not form crowded clusters and may be extremely few and dispersed throughout the smear. Since cancer cells may surround and mingle with normal breast ducts, it is possible to be misled by the presence of completely benign ductal layers with rare single tumor cells in the background. Thus, isolated atypical cells must not be ignored. Lobular carcinoma is often a highly fibrotic and poorly cellular lesion. Thus, cellularity in the cytological smear may be scarce, and the aspirate could be inadequate. For these reasons, the false-negative rate in FNA of lobular carcinomas is high (8–22%) [Abdulla et al., 2000; Robinson et al., 1995].

Lobular carcinoma cells are typically small in size (10–15 μm) with a very high nuclear/cytoplasmic ratio. They are isolated and dispersed, or are grouped together in small and poorly cohesive clusters with occasional alignments of single cells [Menet et al., 2007]. Nuclei are round or mildly dysmorphic, with homogeneously distributed and finely granular chromatin. The cytoplasm is light and may contain mucin vacuoles, sometimes with a small dense stain in the center that gives the cell the characteristic "target-like appearance" (Fig. 9). This vacuole may compress and indent the nucleus or push it at the periphery of the cell, defining the so-called "signet-ring cells." Signet-ring cells are often present in lobular carcinomas but only rarely represent the majority of the cancer cell population [Tsuchiya, 2008].

Aspirates from lobular carcinomas of the pleomorphic variant may display markedly atypical cells with evident nucleoli, mitotic figures, and larger, indented, and budding nuclei. These neoplasms are difficult to recognize as lobular on cytology and are usually diagnosed as moderately or poorly differentiated ductal carcinomas NST (Fig. 10).

Summary

Key Cytological Features of Lobular Carcinoma

- Scarce and scattered cellularity
- Small, monomorphic cells
- Isolated cells or poorly cohesive clusters; occasional alignments of single cells (Indian files)
- Round, mildly irregular, nuclear contours; homogeneous and finely granular chromatin
- Inconspicuous nucleoli
- Cytoplasmic vacuoles with targetoid appearance, occasional signet-ring features

Common Pitfalls of FNA: Lobular Carcinoma

- Scarce cellularity
- Mild atypia
- Small nuclei, similar to those of normal cells or histiocytes
- Presence of benign ductal cell layers

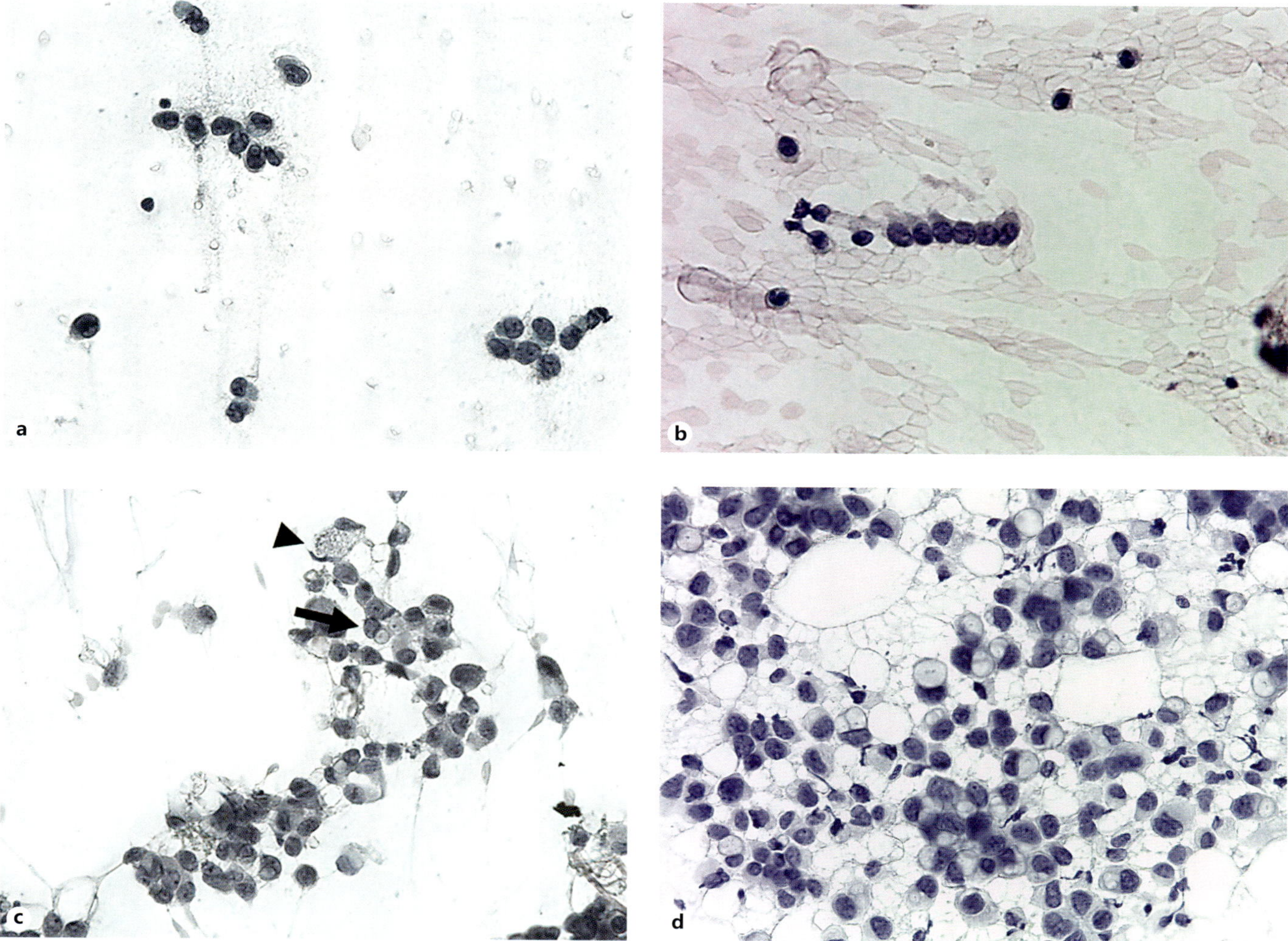

Fig. 9. Cytology of lobular carcinoma. Aspirates from lobular carcinomas are often scarcely cellular, displaying a population of dispersed, small, neoplastic cells with high nuclear/cytoplasmic ratio and vesicular nuclei (**a**), which may sometimes be arranged in short Indian files (**b**). The cytoplasm is commonly occupied by a single mucin vacuole containing a central dot of dense material (arrow) (**c**). Note the difference with the microvacuolated cytoplasm of foamy cells (arrowhead) (**c**). The cytoplasmic vacuole may be prominent, pushing the nucleus at the periphery of the cell and giving the "signet-ring-cell" aspect (**d**). Papanicolaou. High power.

Tubular Carcinoma

Introduction/Epidemiology

Tubular carcinoma is a specific type with a particularly favorable prognosis accounting for approximately 2% of all invasive cancers and presenting almost always at an early stage as a small, spiculated, mammographic opacity (Fig. 11). It can be multifocal in approximately 10–20% of cases and is seen at ultrasound as a hypoechoic lesion with ill-defined margins and posterior acoustic shadowing [Sheppard et al., 2000].

Histological Features

Tubular carcinoma is composed of well-differentiated tubular structures with open lumina lined by a single layer of cells in a fibrous and desmoplastic stroma (Fig. 12). The cells are small to moderate in size and rather monomorphic, with small, inconspicuous nucleoli and scanty mitotic figures. Many well- or moderately differentiated ductal carcinoma NST may show some sort of tubular differentiation without being classified as tubular carcinomas. Actually, there is a lack of consensus concerning the proportion of tubular structures necessary to classify a tumor as tubular carcino-

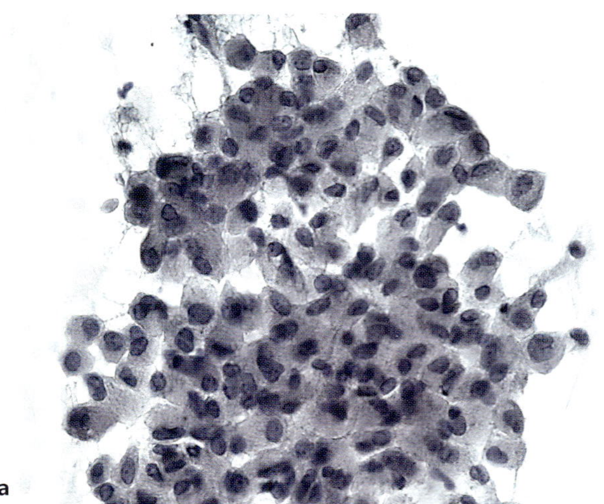

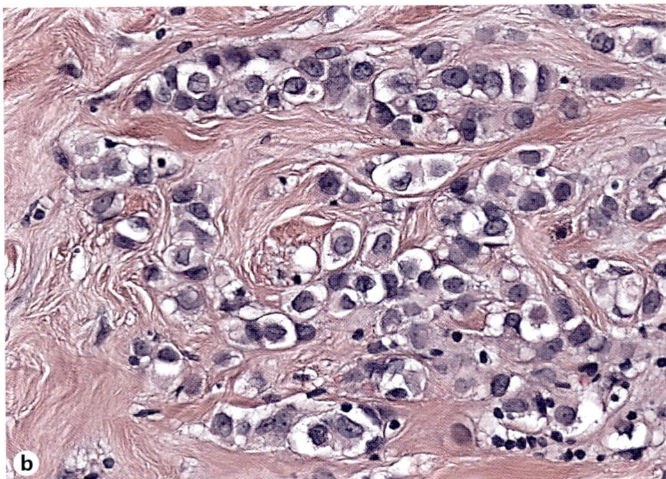

Fig. 10. Pleomorphic variant of lobular carcinoma. Cancer cells are arranged in clusters and show irregular nuclear shapes and a wide amount of granular (apocrine) cytoplasm (**a**). These are unusual features for a lobular carcinoma, and the only clue that might give a hint to the nature of these cells is the quality of nuclear chromatin. This case was assessed as "carcinoma" (C5), and the correct diagnosis was made on the histological section after immunostaining for E-cadherin. Papanicolaou (**a**) and H&E (**b**). High power.

ma, with the requirements being set between 75 and 100% [Lakhani et al., 2012].

Tubular carcinoma is almost always positive for hormonal receptors and negative for HER2 [Papadatos et al., 2001].

Cytology
Since this neoplasm shares many morphological features with well-differentiated invasive ductal carcinoma, it is not possible to make a definite diagnosis of tubular carcinoma on the cytological specimen. It is still possible to suspect and suggest this neoplasm in the presence of a monomorphic population of slightly atypical cells arranged in cohesive tubular aggregates lacking myoepithelial cells, assessing it as "well-differentiated carcinoma" or "suspicious for carcinoma" if the radiological findings are discordant. The tubular clusters have a peculiar angular or "comma-like" appearance and very neat borders, but myoepithelial cells and bare nuclei are missing or are extremely few. Some scattered isolated cells with intact cytoplasm may be present, and the background is typically clean (Fig. 13).

The high cohesiveness of cellular aggregates and minimal cytological atypia put this lesion in the differential diagnosis with some benign proliferative lesions, such as sclerosing adenosis and fibroadenomas (Fig. 14). The radiological appearance of a spiculated mass is usually sufficient to suggest the presence of this lesion to the cytopathologist. Then, a careful analysis of nuclear polarization in the clusters, together with the absence of myoepithelial cells and bare bipolar nuclei allow to correctly assess the specimen as malignant.

Summary
Key Cytological Features of Tubular Carcinoma
- Moderate to marked cellularity
- Highly cohesive tubular aggregates of monomorphic cells with angular shapes and neat borders
- Absence of myoepithelial cells
- Clean background

Common Pitfalls of FNA: Tubular Carcinoma
- Very mild cytological atypia
- Occasional myoepithelial cells or bare nuclei

Mucinous Carcinoma

Introduction/Epidemiology
Mucinous carcinoma (also known as colloid or gelatinous carcinoma) accounts for 1–6% of all breast carcinomas [Di

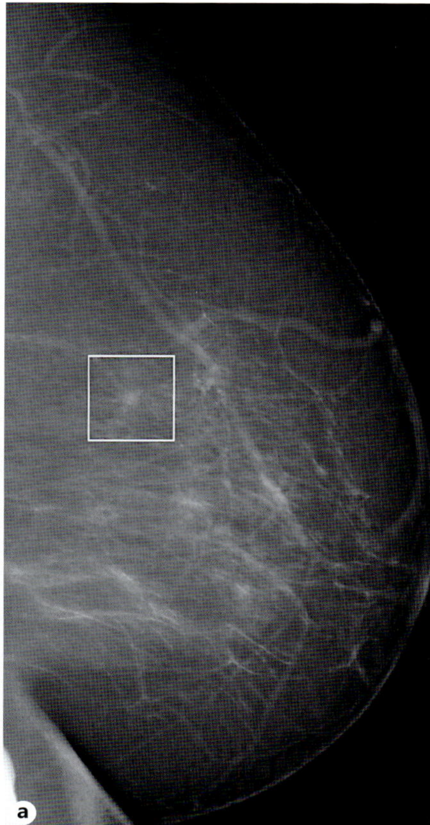

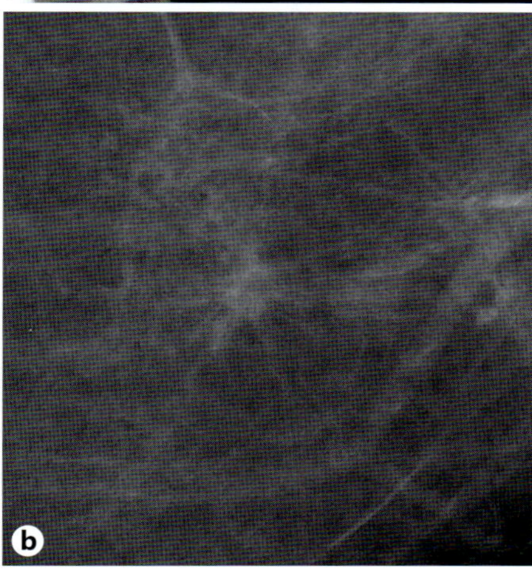

Fig. 11. Mammogram of tubular carcinoma. This lesion is visible as a small, stellate opacity in the upper-outer quadrant of the right breast (**a**). Such a small lesion can be difficult to detect, but the spiculated contours, better appreciated at higher magnification, are highly suspicious (**b**).

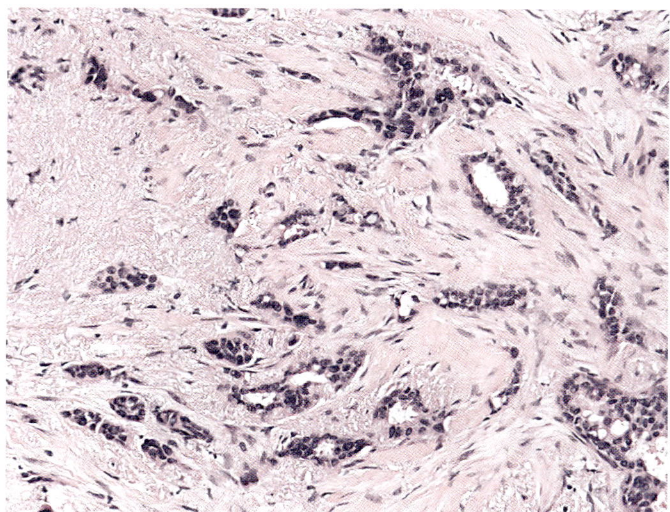

Fig. 12. Histology of tubular carcinoma. The neoplasm is composed of small tubular structures lined by a single layer of cuboidal cells with bland nuclei and without myoepithelial cells in a desmoplastic stroma. H&E. Low power.

Saverio et al., 2008]. Its pure form, which represents less than 2% of breast cancers, is known to have a very good prognosis, while the mixed form, in which a nonmucinous invasive pattern is present, carries a worse prognosis, comparable to that of patients with ductal carcinoma NST [Toikkanen et al., 1988]. Mucinous carcinoma usually presents in elderly postmenopausal women and gives rarely origin to lymph node or distant metastases. Macroscopically, it is well circumscribed and has a peculiar soft/gelatinous consistence, which could make the clinical diagnosis less reliable. Mammography and ultrasound highlight the neoplasm as a mass with well-circumscribed, round or lobular shape, or may show a less-defined, irregular mass in mixed tumors [Zhang et al., 2015].

Histological Features

Pure mucinous carcinomas can be subdivided into *cellular* and *hypocellular* variants based on the degree of cellularity and the architectural pattern. The hypocellular variant shows a tubular, cribriform, cord-like, micropapillary, or papillary growth pattern, while the cellular variant grows in solid nests (Fig. 15). Tumors with a predominantly papillary pattern tend to be more aggressive and tend to more frequently show axillary lymph node metastases at diagnosis than other pure mucinous carcinomas [Ranade et al., 2010]. The tumor cells in pure mucinous carcinomas typically show mild pleomorphism.

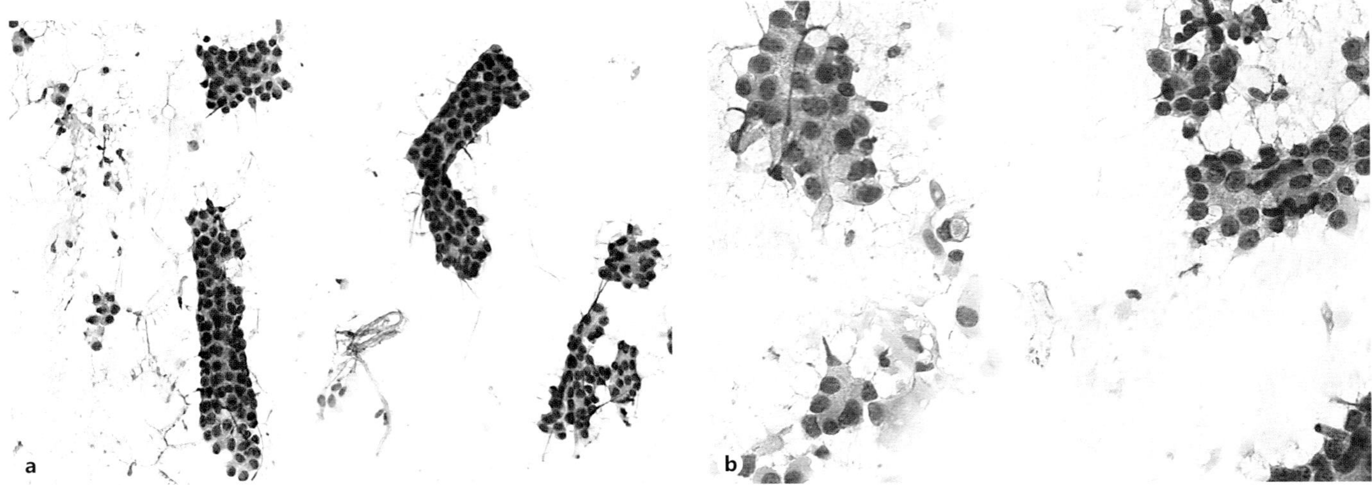

Fig. 13. Cytology of tubular carcinoma. This aspirate displays numerous medium-sized tubular aggregates of monomorphic cancer cells with round to oval-shaped nuclei in a clean background. Tubular clusters have neat borders but lack myoepithelial cells (**a**). Scattered intact cells occasionally show cytoplasmic vacuoles (**b**). Papanicolaou. **a** Intermediate power. **b** High power.

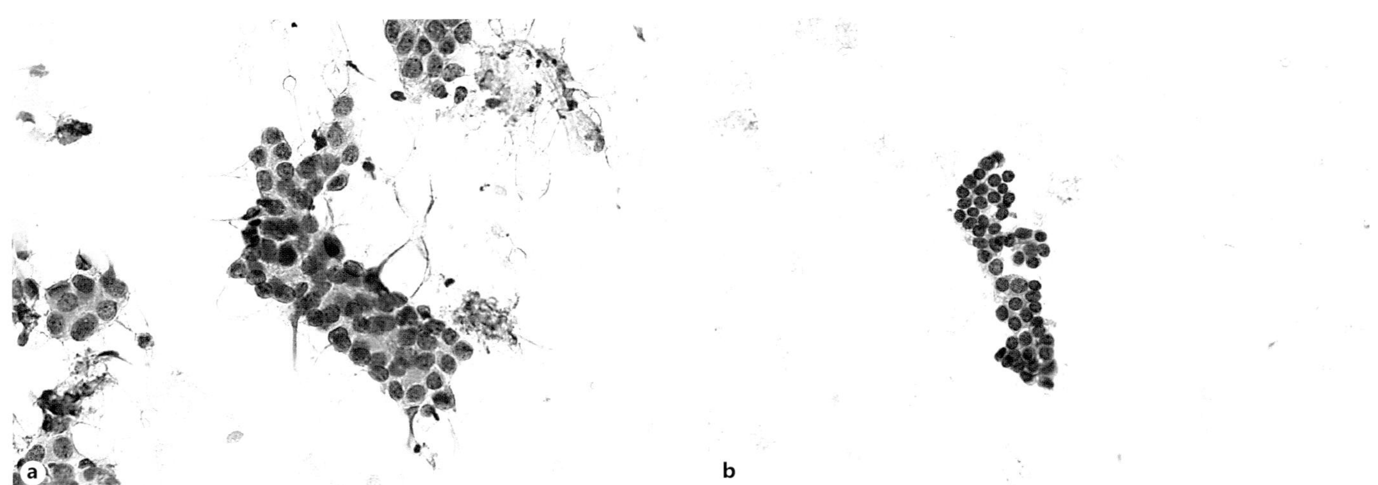

Fig. 14. Differential diagnosis between tubular carcinoma (**a**) and sclerosing adenosis (**b**). Well-differentiated carcinomas share many cytological features with some benign ductal lesions. These 2 cases are depicted at the same magnification. Note the increased nuclear size and the "railway-track" aspect with rigid borders of the tubular cluster in the first lesion (**a**) compared with those of the second one (**b**). Myoepithelial cells are not evident in any of the 2 cases. Papanicolaou. High power.

A significant portion of pure mucinous carcinomas shows neuroendocrine differentiation, which can be suspected histologically based on morphological features such as an insular or solid pattern, stippled chromatin, and a general "uniformity" of cancer cells. The confirmation of the neuroendocrine nature of cancer cells comes from immunohistochemistry, with cancer cells positive for one or more of the so-called "neuroendocrine markers" (chromogranin A, synaptophysin, neuron-specific enolase, and/or CD56). Neuroendocrine differentiation can be seen in many subtypes of breast cancer, but it is most common in pure mucinous carcinomas. Its significance in clinical practice has still not been well established, but a recent study identified the neuroendocrine variant of mucinous carcinoma as a tumor occurring later in life, with a low nuclear grade, favorable immunohistochemical features, and a lower rate of distant metastases at diagnosis [Tse et al., 2004].

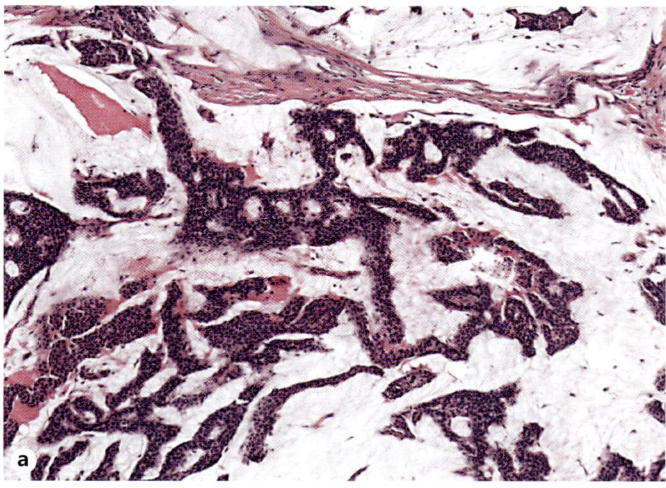

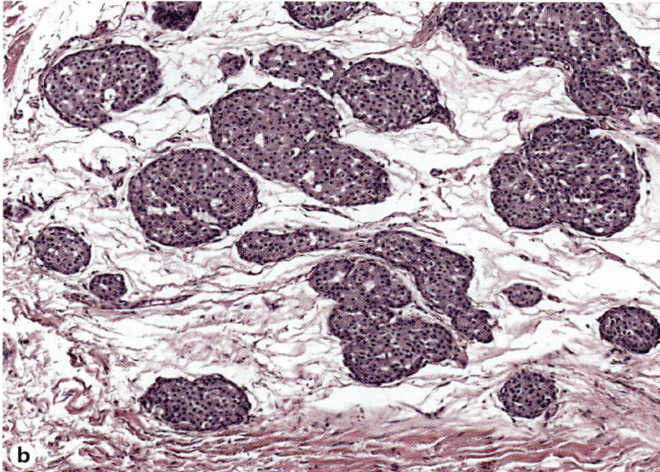

Fig. 15. Histology of mucinous carcinoma. The *hypocellular* variant of mucinous carcinoma may show a cribriform and cord-like growth pattern (**a**), while the *cellular* variant has a predominantly solid pattern (**b**). In both variants, the neoplastic cell component is immersed in abundant extracellular mucin. H&E. Low power.

Pure mucinous carcinomas are frequently (96%) estrogen (ER)/progesterone receptor (PR) positive and HER-2 negative [Kashiwagi et al., 2013].

Cytology

Despite its slight cytological atypia, FNAC is highly accurate in identifying mucinous carcinomas, even though the definitive distinction between the pure and mixed form is unreliable cytopathologically [Cyrta et al., 2013]. The most important and peculiar aspect of aspirates taken from mucinous carcinomas is the presence of extracellular mucin, which may be evident macroscopically as a translucent, slimy, and gelatinous substance that tends to dry quickly after the smear. On microscopical evaluation, mucus appears as a background gray to green-bluish transparent film in Pap-stained preparations or blue to magenta amorphous substance in Giemsa-stained preparations. Cancer cells are arranged singly or in 3-dimensional clusters with smooth borders and sometimes with evident micropapillary outline (Fig. 16). They are quite monomorphic, with plasmacytoid appearance, small nuclei (less than 2 times a red blood cell), regular nuclear membrane, and inconspicuous nucleoli. Myoepithelial cells are absent, as well as bare bipolar nuclei in the background, which is dominated by mucous substance and isolated cancer cells. Some thin-walled branching ("chicken wire") vessels might be present in the mucus, and they are fairly typical of mucinous carcinomas although not exclusive.

The finding of features such as necrosis (typically absent in pure mucinous carcinomas), large nuclei (more than 3 times a red blood cell), irregular nuclear outlines, evident nucleoli, or a scarce amount of mucin (<25%) are highly suggestive of the presence of a mixed tumor [Cyrta et al., 2013].

A neuroendocrine nature can be suspected on the cytological sample in the presence of intracytoplasmic granules in a monotonous population of plasmacytoid cells with low-grade atypia and inconspicuous nucleoli, but we do not recommend making this diagnosis based on morphology alone. In contrast to neuroendocrine carcinomas of other organs, neuroendocrine carcinomas of the breast uncommonly present the classical "salt-and-pepper" chromatin pattern [Ohashi et al., 2016].

A differential diagnosis between mucinous carcinomas and mucocele-like lesions or myxoid fibroadenoma may be difficult based on cytology due to the low-grade nuclear atypia of this neoplasm. Close attention must be paid to cellular cohesion, which is usually maintained in mucocele lesions and fibroadenomas and easily lost in mucinous carcinomas, and to the presence of myoepithelial cells and bare bipolar nuclei [Ventura et al., 2003].

In everyday clinical practice, we recommend the use of the term "carcinoma with features of mucinous differentiation," since even cases with all the typical features of pure mucinous carcinoma might have been partially sampled and might result as mixed tumors on the definitive histological specimen due to intratumor heterogeneity.

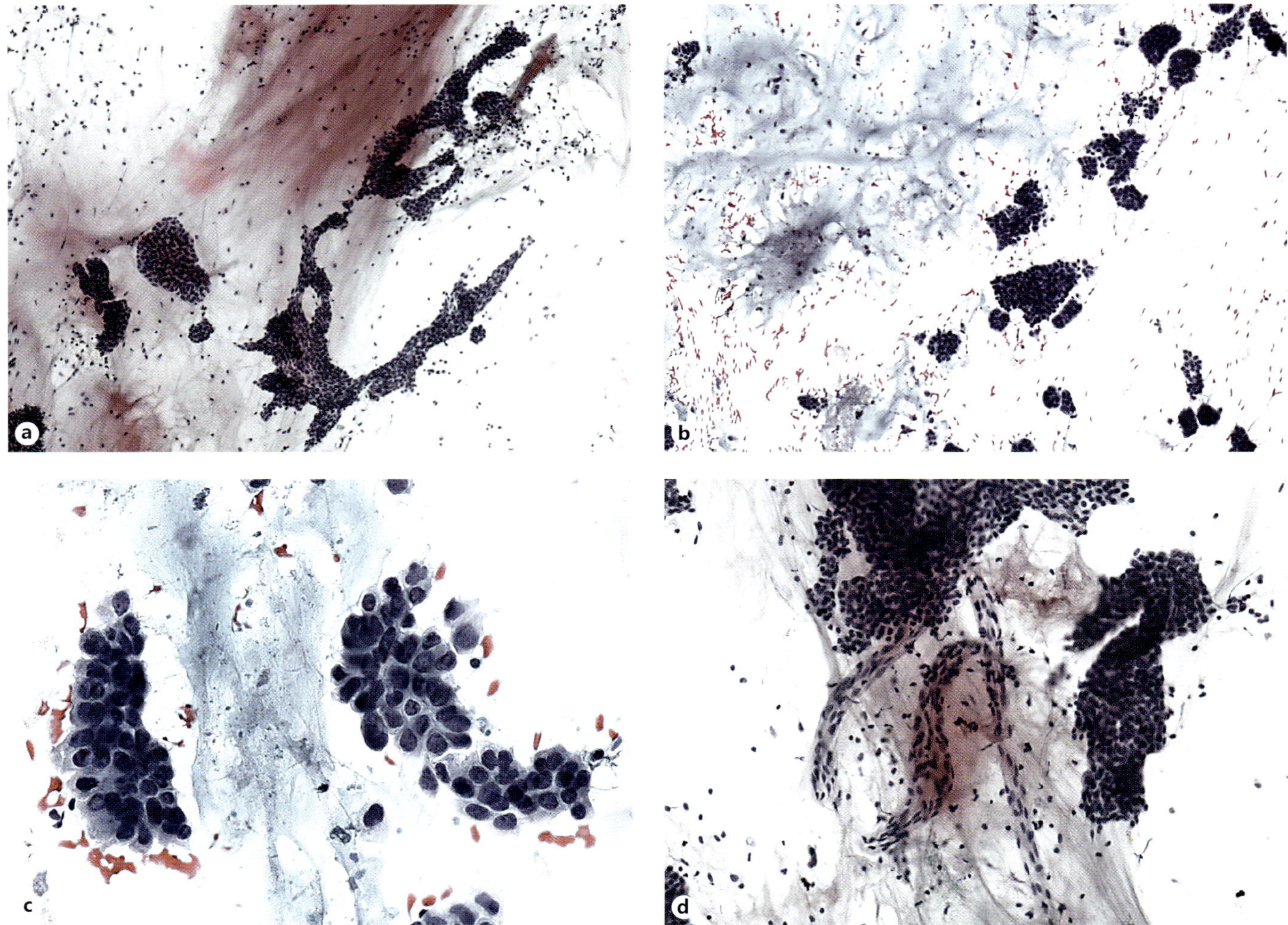

Fig. 16. Cytology of mucinous carcinoma. Aspirates from mucinous carcinomas typically show cancer cells with low-grade to moderate atypia arranged singly and in clusters in a myxoid background. Extracellular mucin may appear bluish or pink-purple in Pap-stained preparations (**a**, **b**). At higher magnification, cancer cell clusters show smooth borders and lack myoepithelial cells (**c**). Thin-walled, branching vessels might be visible in the myxoid background creating the image of a "chicken wire" (**d**). Papanicolaou. **a**, **b**, **d** Low power. **c** High power.

Summary

Key Cytological Features of Mucinous Carcinoma

- Abundant extracellular mucin
- Cancer cells with small nuclei and regular nuclear membranes
- Three-dimensional clusters without myoepithelial cells
- Absence of nucleoli
- Thin-walled, "chicken wire" vessels

Common Pitfalls of FNA: Mucinous Carcinoma

- Mild nuclear atypia
- Presence of more atypical cells and nonmucinous component (mixed type)
- Mucin-like extracellular substance in nonmucinous lesions (myxoid fibroadenoma)

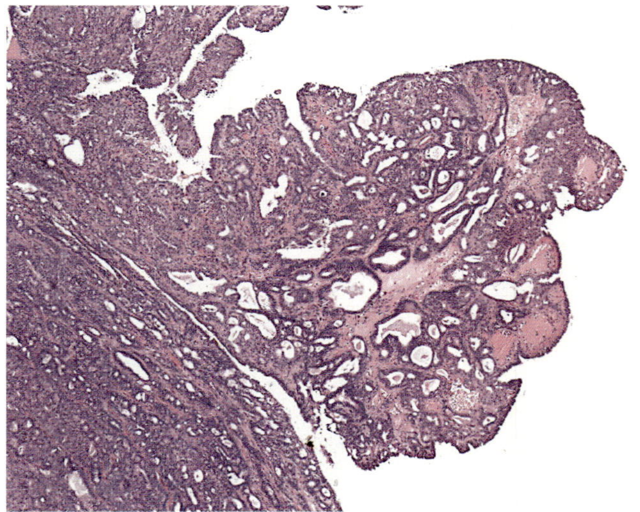

Fig. 17. Histology of papillary carcinoma. This partially cystic lesion shows complex branching papillary stalks lined by relatively monomorphic cancer cells. A clearly invasive component is present in the left lower part of the picture. Myoepithelial cells are not present, neither in the papillary nor in the invasive component. H&E. Low power.

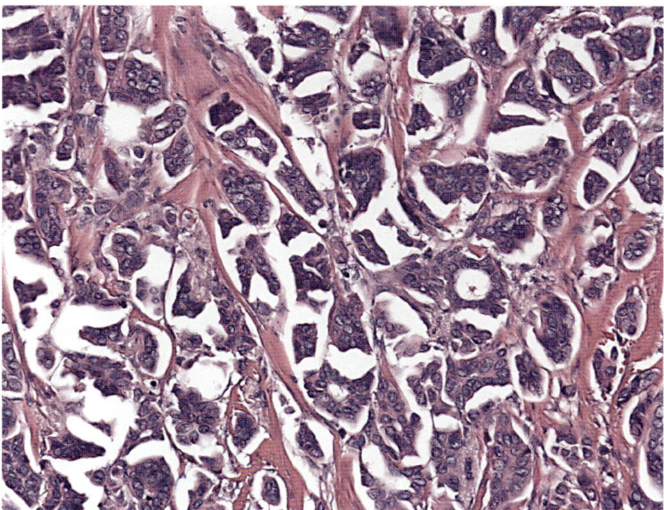

Fig. 18. Micropapillary carcinoma. Neoplastic cells are arranged in small morula-like clusters with central pseudolumina, devoid of fibrovascular cores, and surrounded by artifacts of stromal spaces. H&E. High power.

Papillary Carcinoma

Introduction/Epidemiology

Pure papillary carcinoma of the breast is a rare tumor affecting predominantly elderly postmenopausal women and has a favorable prognosis, accounting for 0.3–2% of all breast malignancies [Fisher et al., 1980]. The so-called *encapsulated* or *intracystic* papillary carcinoma is defined by the presence of papillary carcinoma within a cystically dilated duct and surrounded by a fibrous capsule. It has indolent behavior and rarely metastasizes. Papillary carcinomas are often located near the areola and may thus present as palpable masses or nipple discharge. Imaging findings of papillary carcinomas may overlap with those of benign papillary lesions or might infrequently show signs of a more obvious infiltration of the breast tissue, similarly to ductal carcinoma NST. Papillary carcinoma is more common in the male than the female breast [Reid-Nicholson et al., 2006].

Histological Features

The lesion is composed of complex branching fibrovascular cores lined by epithelial cells that usually show mild or moderate atypia (Fig. 17). The absence of an intact myoepithelial cell layer within papillary structures is an important marker to define these lesions. A papillary component may be found in association with DCIS or invasive ductal carcinoma NST.

Pure papillary carcinomas are well-differentiated neoplasms (grade 1 or 2) that usually express hormonal receptors and are negative for HER2/neu.

Invasive *micropapillary* carcinoma is an aggressive variant composed of small, morula-like clusters of cuboidal to columnar cancer cells devoid of fibrovascular cores and surrounded by clear stromal spaces (Fig. 18). It is an uncommon pure type with a tendency to vascular invasion and higher stage at diagnosis. Compared with other papillary neoplasms and with invasive ductal carcinoma NST, micropapillary carcinomas are more frequently HER2 positive [Walsh and Bleiweiss, 2001].

Cytology

As mentioned before in Chapter 6 [this vol., pp. 41–57], it is very difficult and sometimes impossible to distinguish benign from malignant papillary lesions on a cytological smear. In addition, the differentiation between noninvasive intraductal papillary carcinoma and frankly invasive papillary carcinoma is problematic due to identical cytological features [Simsir et al., 2002].

Features like marked cellularity, complex branching papillary fragments, and single atypical intact cells have been

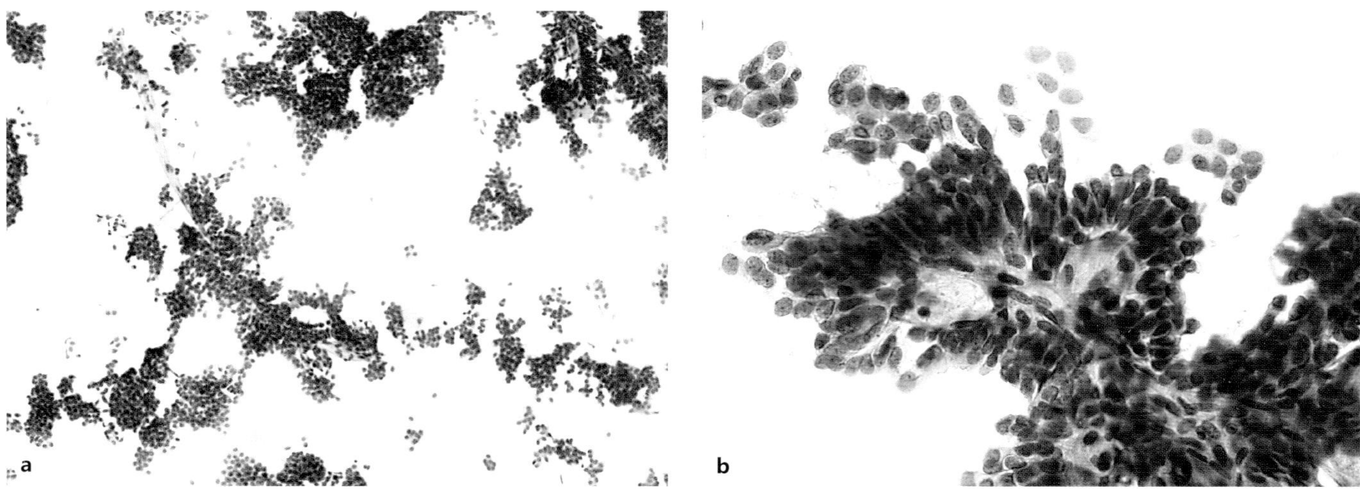

Fig. 19. Cytology of papillary carcinoma. This markedly cellular smear shows several complex and branching clusters with a stromal and an epithelial component and numerous dissociated epithelial cells. Cell clusters are hypercellular, vary widely in size and shape, and lack myoepithelial elements. Similarly, bare bipolar nuclei are relatively rare compared to the epithelial cylindrical cells with intact cytoplasm. Papanicolaou. **a** Low power. **b** High power.

suggested to point toward the malignant nature of the tumor (Fig. 19, 20) [Dawson and Mulford, 1994]. However, these features have not been found to be restricted to malignant lesions [Simsir et al., 2003]. Other features that should be examined and that could orient toward malignancy include the absence of bland columnar cells and lack of foamy or hemosiderin-laden macrophages in the background, as well as the absence of myoepithelial cells in the papillary clusters.

Sometimes the malignant nature of a lesion is more obvious, but it is still difficult to address the tumor as papillary carcinoma or any other type of carcinoma. Invasive ductal carcinoma with focal papillary areas usually shows highly cellular smears with complex crowded epithelial cell sheets displaying higher nuclear atypia and irregularities. Bare nuclei in the background are usually absent.

Micropapillary carcinoma lacks true fibrovascular cores and shows numerous well-formed angular and morular clusters of small- to medium-sized atypical cells (Fig. 21) [Khurana et al., 1997].

Distinguishing papillary carcinoma from benign papillary lesions of the breast is extremely important, and there is still an open debate about the management of papillary lesions identified by biopsy or cytology [Prathiba et al., 2010]. Much attention must be paid to the presence or absence of cytological atypia. Neither FNAC nor core needle biopsy is able to exclude malignancy with absolute certainty, and carcinoma foci have been found in 2.3% of the excised papillary lesions with pathological and radiological findings indicating a benign nature [Pareja et al., 2016]. Nevertheless, we agree that this percentage is too low to justify surgical excision in all cases of papillary lesions and suggest close radiological and cytological follow-up in women without atypia in the cytological sample and without additional risk factors. Conversely, the presence of cytological findings suspicious of malignancy, cytological-radiological discordance, or individual risk factors, such as a family history of breast cancer or the presence of predisposing genetic mutations, should lead to surgical excision.

Summary

Key Cytological Features of Papillary Carcinoma

- Marked cellularity
- Complex branching papillary clusters without myoepithelial cells
- Isolated atypical intact cells (not bare nuclei)

Common Pitfalls of FNA: Papillary Carcinoma

- Bland atypia
- Papillary component admixed with nonpapillary malignant clusters

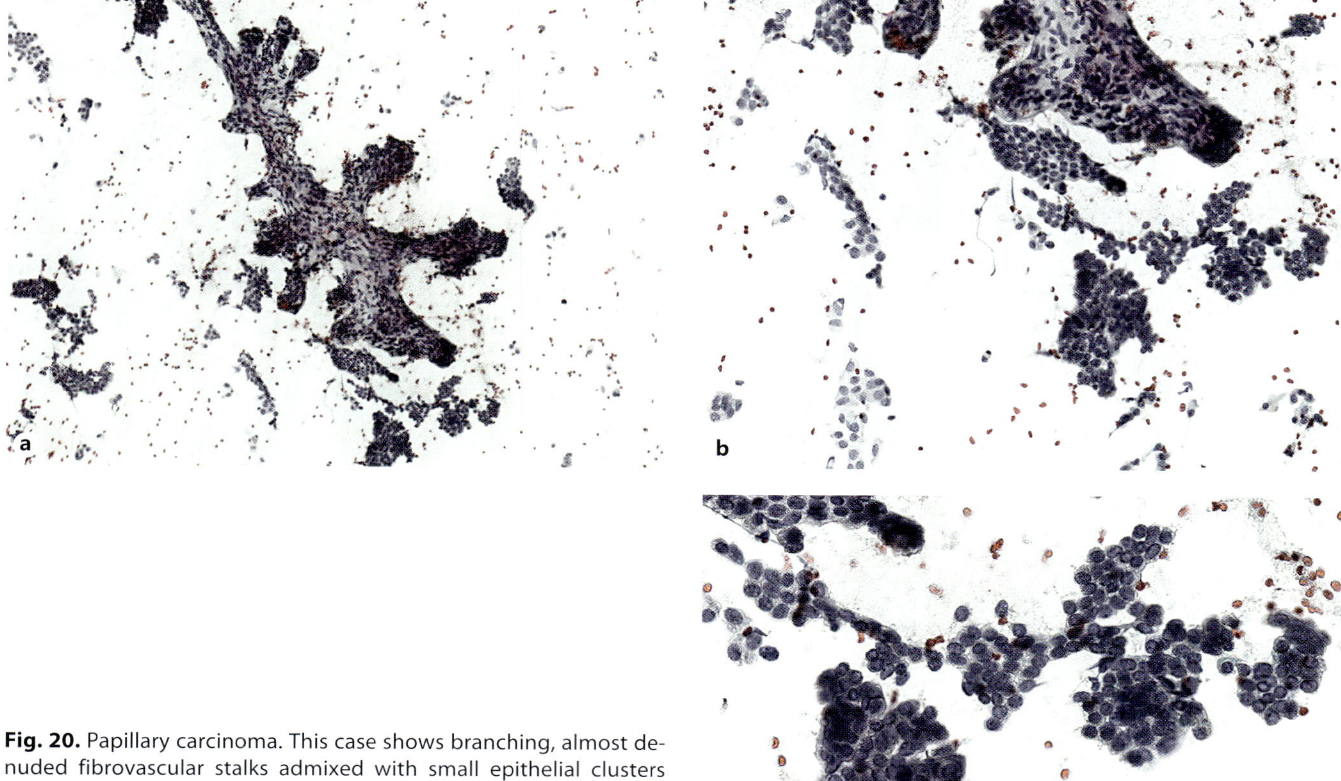

Fig. 20. Papillary carcinoma. This case shows branching, almost denuded fibrovascular stalks admixed with small epithelial clusters composed of monotonous round cells (**a**, **b**). Cytological atypia is low, but nuclei are densely packed, and myoepithelial cells are not present (**c**). This case was diagnosed as papillary proliferation with atypia, suspicious for papillary carcinoma (C4) and referred to histology for a definite diagnosis. An invasive papillary carcinoma was diagnosed on the surgical specimen. Papanicolaou. **a** Low power. **b** Intermediate power. **c** High power.

Carcinoma with Medullary Features

Introduction/Epidemiology

Formerly known as medullary carcinoma, it is a rare subtype of invasive breast cancer characterized by neat borders, lymphocyte-rich stroma, marked cytological atypia, and a relatively good prognosis compared with invasive ductal carcinoma NST. This neoplasm predominantly occurs in middle-aged women, but it can also be found in younger patients, since it is frequently associated with BRCA1 germline mutations [Eisinger et al., 1998]. Mammography and ultrasonography usually show a well-defined mass, which is typically soft on clinical examination.

Histological Features

The neoplasm is composed of markedly atypical epithelial cells with large, pleomorphic nuclei and prominent nucleoli, which do not form glandular structures and grow in solid nests with syncytial features. Abundant inflammatory infiltrate composed mainly of lymphocytes surrounds and permeates the tumor, clearly demarcating the neoplasm from normal breast parenchyma (Fig. 22). Foci of DCIS as well as lobular neoplasm around the tumor are uncommon findings.

Despite the presence of markedly atypical cells, which are typically ER, PR, and HER2 negative, when properly diagnosed following strict criteria, carcinoma with medullary features has a good prognosis, with low rates of lymph node or distant metastases [Pedersen et al., 1995].

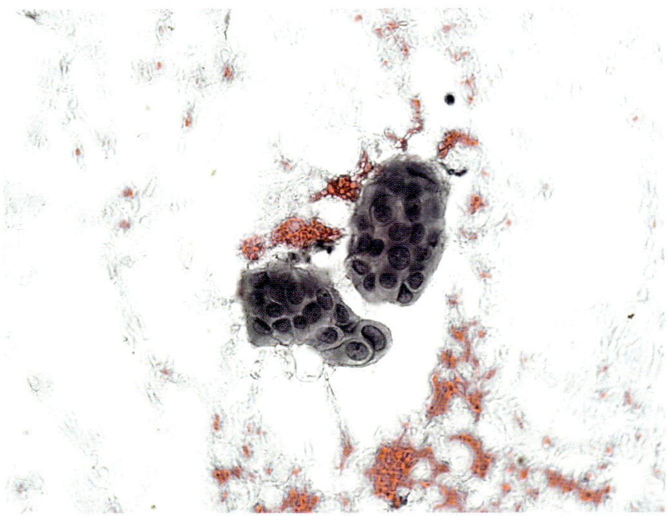

Fig. 21. Cytology of micropapillary carcinoma. The hallmarks of this lesion are small morula-like clusters with smooth margins composed of epithelial cells with round and relatively bland nuclei. These clusters lack myoepithelial cells and fibrovascular stalks. Papanicolaou. High power.

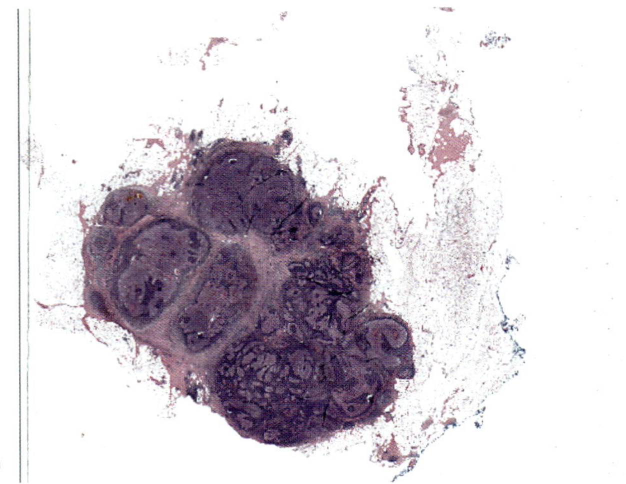

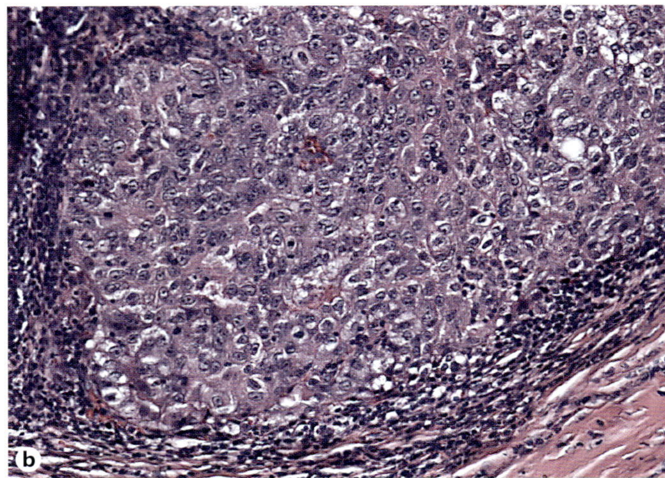

Fig. 22. Histology of carcinoma with medullary features. This neoplasm is defined as a lesion with the following histological features: solid architecture, pushing borders (**a**), rich lymphocytic intratumor infiltrate, high nuclear grade, and syncytial growth pattern (**b**). Note that lymphocytes are present also in the cytoplasm of cancer cells. H&E. **a** Slide overview. **b** High power.

Cytology

Aspirates from carcinomas with medullary features usually produce hypercellular smears with a variable admixture of markedly atypical cancer cells and chronic inflammatory cells. Neoplastic cells show one or more large pleomorphic nuclei, prominent nucleoli, and more than occasional mitotic figures, and are arranged singly or in 3-dimensional and loosely cohesive clusters (Fig. 23, 24). Tubular or acinar aggregates are typically absent, since the neoplasm has a solid-syncytial growth pattern. Many lymphocytes and plasma cells are admixed with neoplastic cells, and the background is necrotic [Galzerano et al., 2014].

A diagnosis of malignancy based on FNAC is usually easy, but it is important to differentiate this tumor from other more aggressive neoplasms in order to provide the patients with the best treatment. The presence of duct-like aggregates of cancer cells should orient the diagnosis towards ductal carcinoma NST rather than medullary carcinoma regardless of the lymphocytic infiltrate. Note that the definition of carcinoma with medullary features includes neat borders and clear circumscription of the neoplasm; therefore, a cytological diagnosis cannot be made without a careful radiological evaluation.

A large cell lymphoma could be suspected based on the aspirate, but the distinct nature of the large pleomorphic cells and the small reactive lymphocytes are usually sufficiently clear based on morphology. In selected cases, immunocytochemical stains for CD45 and cytokeratins may be helpful. Metastatic neoplasms to the breast should also be carefully excluded.

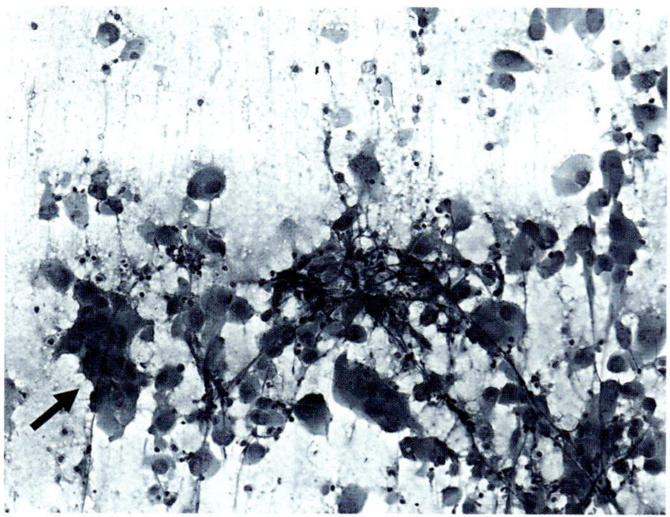

Fig. 23. Cytology of carcinoma with medullary features. A population of markedly atypical, mainly dissociated cancer cells is present in the smear. Some cells are aggregated in syncytial clusters (arrow). The background is dirty, containing cellular debris and many lymphocytes. Papanicolaou. High power.

Summary
Key Cytological Features of Carcinoma with Medullary Features

- Marked cellularity
- Cancer cells with large, pleomorphic, sometimes multiple nuclei, and prominent nucleoli
- Rich lymphocytic infiltrate
- Dirty, necrotic background
- Absence of tubular and acinar structures

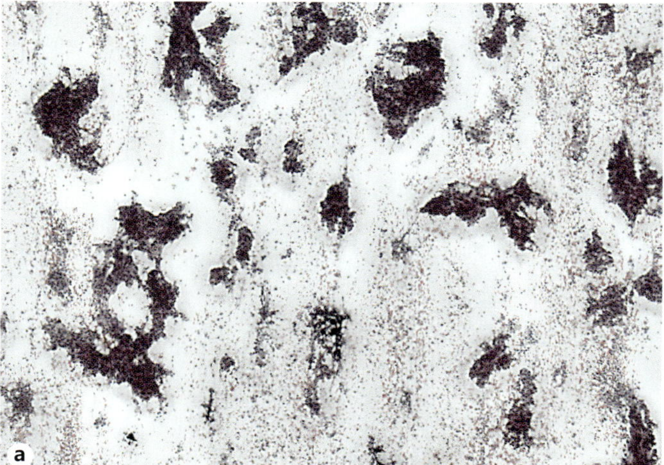

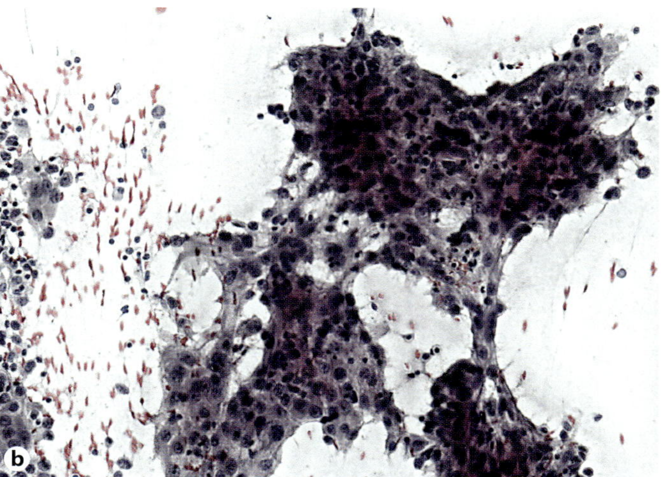

Fig. 24. Medullary carcinoma. This lesion is easily recognized as malignant already on scanning magnification (**a**). Close examination reveals hypercellular clusters of cancer cells with large nuclei, prominent nucleoli, and intracytoplasmic lymphocytes (**b**). The cytological diagnosis was high-grade carcinoma, suspicious for medullary carcinoma (C5). A definite diagnosis of medullary carcinoma is not feasible on cytology, since it relies on specific histological criteria. Papanicolaou. **a** Low power. **b** High power.

Apocrine Carcinoma

Apocrine carcinoma is a rare subtype of breast cancer that can pose diagnostic difficulties based on FNAC due to its morphological aspects resembling those of benign apocrine lesions, from which it must be distinguished. Clinical and radiological aspects are not different from those of invasive ductal carcinoma NST, but some peculiar cytological features can be useful to identify this neoplasm.

Aspirates from invasive apocrine carcinoma usually show numerous, predominantly dispersed, or loosely cohesive epithelial cells with abundant, dense to granular cytoplasm and round to oval nuclei, often eccentrically placed (Fig. 25). Nuclear chromatin is dispersed and a prominent eosinophilic nucleolus is present. Unlike benign apocrine lesions, malignant apocrine lesions show nuclear overlapping, nuclear pleomorphism, a raised nuclear/cytoplasmic ratio, and occasional mitotic figures (Fig. 26) [Khandeparkar et al., 2014]. A dirty, necrotic background is frequently present in aspirates from apocrine carcinomas, while benign lesions tend to show a proteinaceous cystic background with scattered foamy cells. Myoepithelial cells are not useful for this differential diagnosis, because they are frequently absent even in apocrine benign lesions.

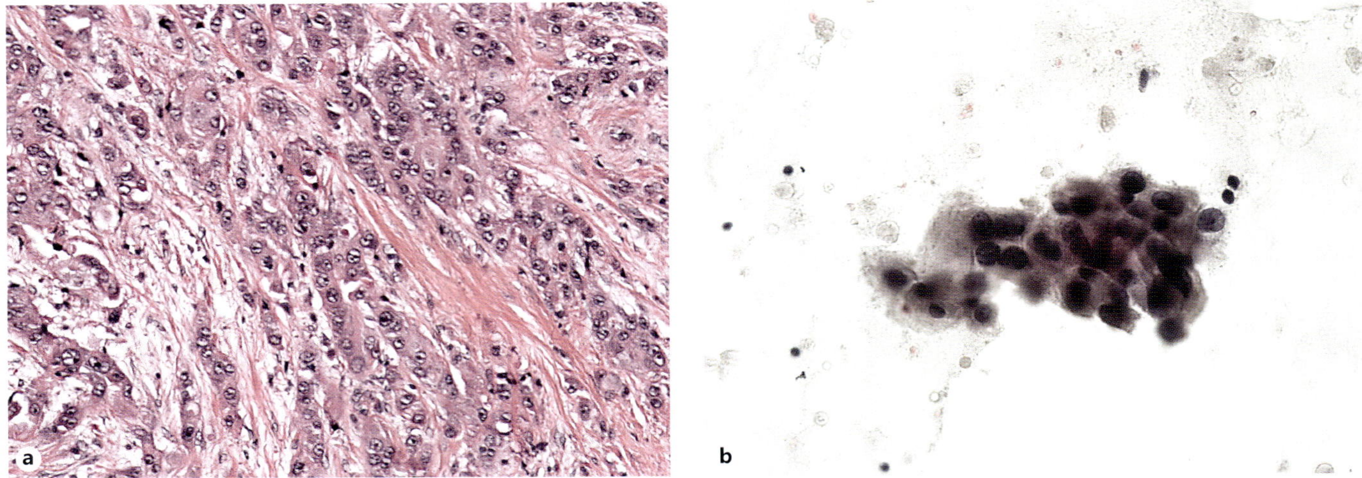

Fig. 25. Apocrine carcinoma. This invasive carcinoma is composed of cells with round nuclei, prominent nucleoli, and granular eosinophilic cytoplasm arranged in sheets and solid nests (**a**). FNAC from the same lesion shows hypercellular clusters with disordered and overlapping nuclei in a dirty background (**b**). H&E (**a**) and Papanicolaou (**b**). **a** Low power. **b** High power.

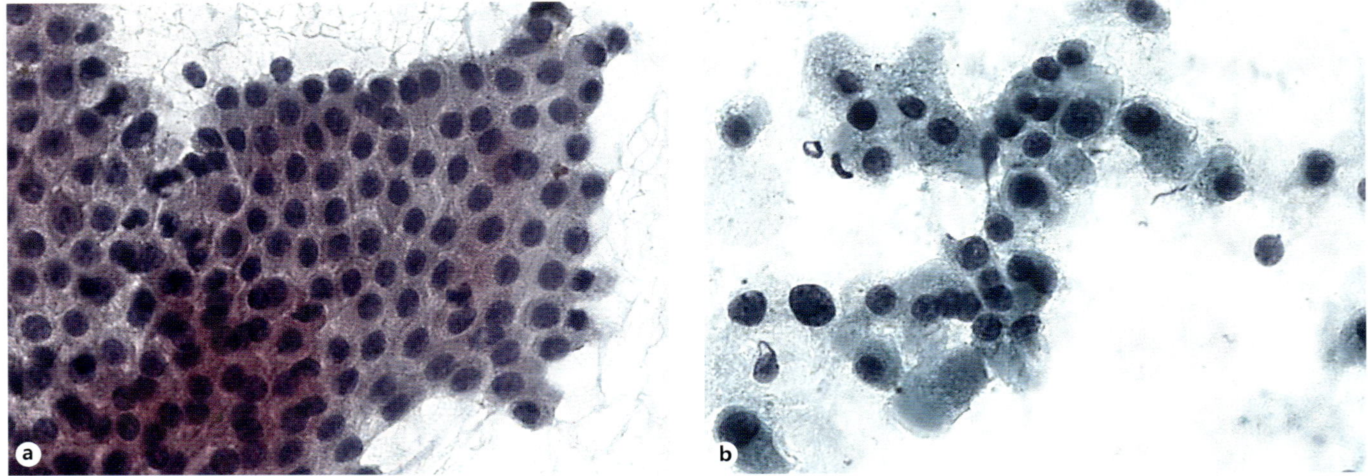

Fig. 26. Differential diagnosis between benign and malignant apocrine lesions. Compared to benign apocrine metaplastic cells (**a**), those of an apocrine carcinoma show greater nuclear pleomorphism and nuclear overlapping, and are arranged in less cohesive, disordered clusters (**b**). Intact single cells are more common in malignant lesions, but they do not represent a reliable sign of malignancy, since they are also present in many benign lesions. Myoepithelial cells, as well as bare bipolar nuclei, are typically lacking in both cases. Papanicolaou. High power.

Secretory Carcinoma

This rare neoplasm is composed of low-grade glandular elements with a solid, tubular, or microcystic architecture and a prominent production of intra- and extracellular secretory material. It may arise in both sexes with a wide age range (3–87 years), being more common in children and young adults [Rosen and Cranor, 1991]. It is more prevalent in the periareolar region and is clinically detected as a well-circumscribed, mobile mass. Histologically, it has pushing borders, and the prognosis is generally good, especially in the younger patients, although it is ER, PR, and HER2/neu negative. These tumors carry a characteristic genetic translocation t(12;15) creating an ETV6-ETRK3 gene fusion, which is considered a very specific diagnostic marker [Lae et al., 2009].

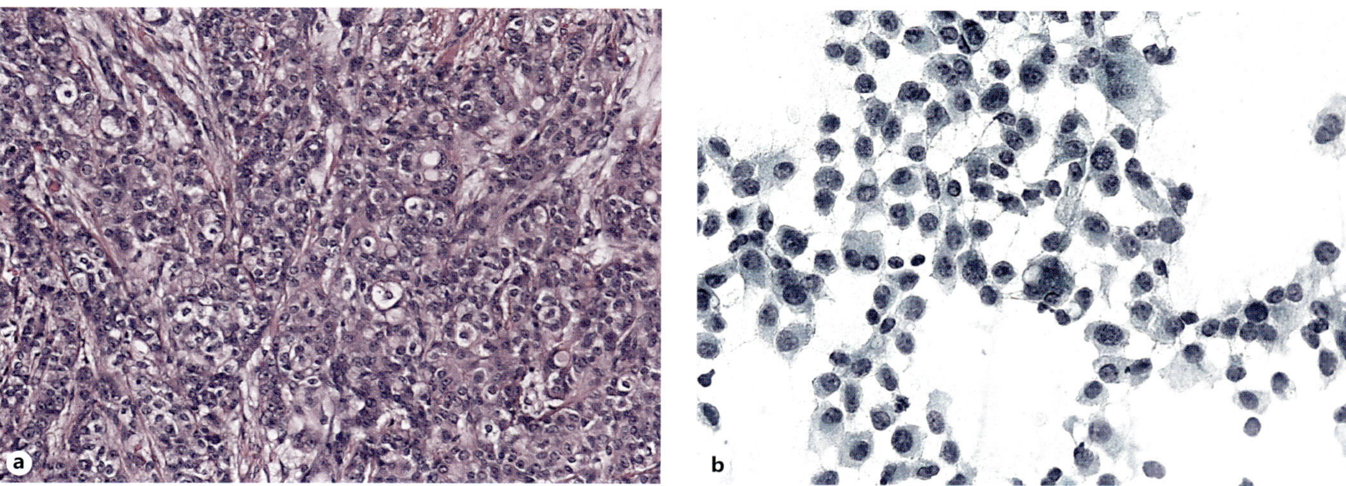

Fig. 27. Secretory carcinoma. This secretory carcinoma shows a predominantly solid architecture and is composed of round and polygonal cells with pale cytoplasm containing secretory vacuoles (**a**). The same cells are well appreciated in the aspirate, where they display singly or in loosely cohesive clusters and show vacuolated or "foamy" cytoplasm (**b**). H&E (**a**) and Papanicolaou (**b**). **a** Low power. **b** High power.

The cytological features of secretory carcinoma can be very similar to those of the normal breast during late pregnancy or lactation, showing clusters of rather uniform epithelial cells with numerous large cytoplasmic vacuoles containing proteinaceous material, which is also present in the background. Nuclei are typically round to oval, with a single, prominent nucleolus and even chromatin (Fig. 27). The absence of myoepithelial cells and bare bipolar nuclei in the background may be a useful diagnostic element to differentiate this neoplasm from lactation changes or a lactating adenoma. Actually, the clinical information is the most important element for this distinction [Vesoulis and Kashkari, 1998].

Metaplastic Carcinoma

Introduction/Epidemiology

Metaplastic carcinoma is a definition used to address a group of invasive carcinomas of the breast characterized by differentiation of the neoplastic cells towards squamous and/or mesenchymal-looking elements, such as spindle, chondroid, osseous, or rhabdomyoid cells. These are rare lesions, accounting for 0.2–5% of all invasive breast carcinomas [Stalsberg and Thomas, 1993]. The age distribution and clinical findings are similar to those of invasive ductal carcinoma NST.

Histological Features

Metaplastic carcinomas are a heterogeneous group of lesions. We find it useful to distinguish some subtypes sharing similar histological features as well as prognostic outcomes (Fig. 28).

The so-called *low-grade adenosquamous carcinomas* are neoplasms composed of well-developed glandular and tubular structures closely admixed with solid nests of squamous cells in a spindle cell background. In some studies, a group of metaplastic carcinomas with a better prognosis and lower risk of distant metastases was identified. Nevertheless, the lesion has a highly infiltrative growth pattern and frequent local recurrences [Van Hoeven et al., 1993].

Fibromatosis-like metaplastic carcinomas are composed of bland-looking spindle cells with slender nuclei and finely distributed chromatin embedded in stroma with varying degree of collagenization. Like the former group, these tumors also seem to have prevalently local aggressiveness, with a generally better prognosis compared to the others [Gobbi et al., 1999].

Pure and mixed *squamous cell carcinomas* of the breast are included among the metaplastic carcinomas. They resemble moderately and poorly differentiated squamous and adenosquamous carcinomas from other organs and have an aggressive behavior. They frequently have central cavitation and may appear as partially cystic masses on ultrasound examination.

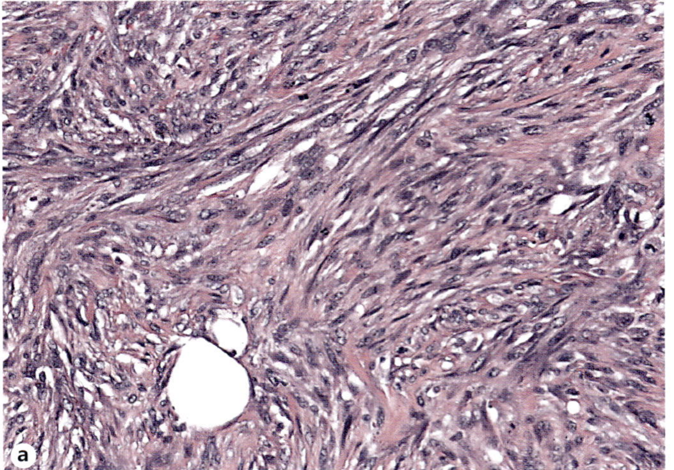

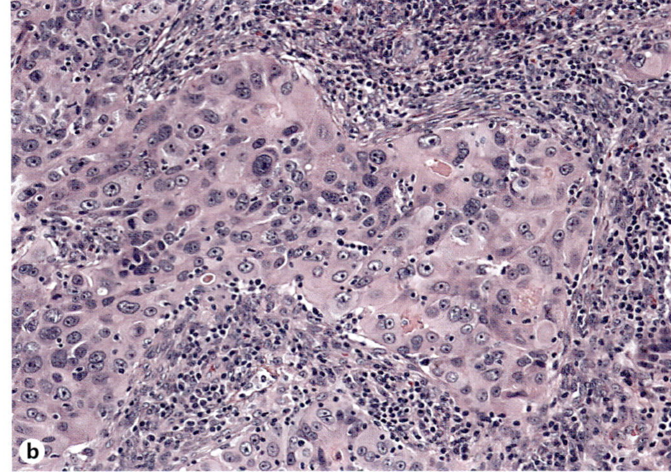

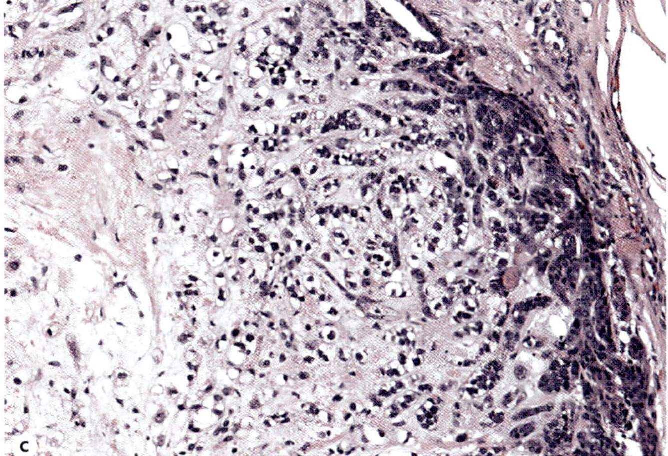

Fig. 28. Metaplastic carcinoma. Metaplastic carcinoma is a heterogeneous entity. Its main histological features include the fibromatosis-like variant (**a**), composed of bundles of spindle cells resembling those of mesenchymal neoplasms, carcinomas with squamous differentiation (**b**), and tumors with heterologous differentiation. **c** A metaplastic carcinoma with chondroid-like stroma. H&E. Intermediate power.

Spindle cell carcinomas are aggressive neoplasms composed of spindle-shaped cells with marked nuclear pleomorphism expressing at least focally epithelial markers (typically p63 and high-molecular-weight cytokeratins).

The last subtype is composed of carcinomas with other uncommon and peculiar mesenchymal differentiations, such as chondroid, osseous, rhabdomyoid, or neuroglial findings. They typically include areas resembling ductal carcinoma NST or squamous cell carcinoma. The term "matrix-producing carcinoma" is reserved to tumors that produce abundant extracellular chondroid matrix.

Metaplastic carcinomas are almost invariably ER, PR and HER2/neu negative [Reis-Filho et al., 2005; Tse et al., 2006].

Cytology

The typical aspirate from a metaplastic carcinoma shows poorly differentiated adenocarcinoma cells arranged singly or in 3-dimensional clusters, admixed with markedly atypical squamous cells, naked carcinomatous nuclei, and necrotic debris (Fig. 29). Pleomorphic spindle cells and chondroid matrix in the background may be present in tumors with mesenchymal differentiation (Fig. 30) [Lale et al., 2011].

Metaplastic carcinomas are known to be potential mimickers of other types of lesions and may represent dangerous pitfalls of cytology depending on the examiner's experience and the type of cells that are present in the smear. Carcinomas with a glandular and a squamous component, and especially low-grade adenosquamous carcinomas, might be only partially sampled, being misdiagnosed as ductal or tu-

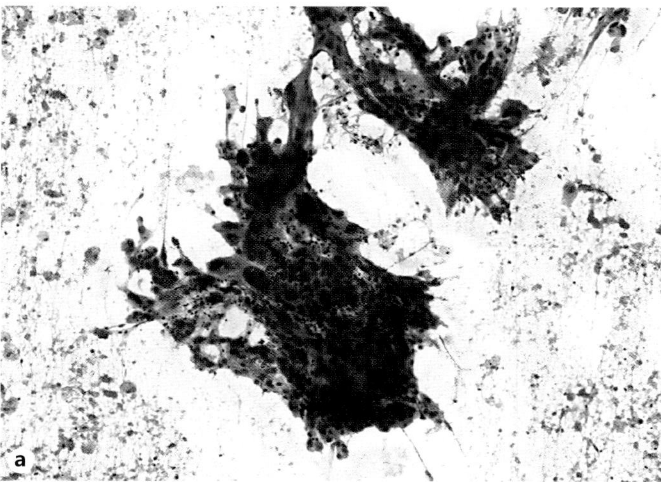

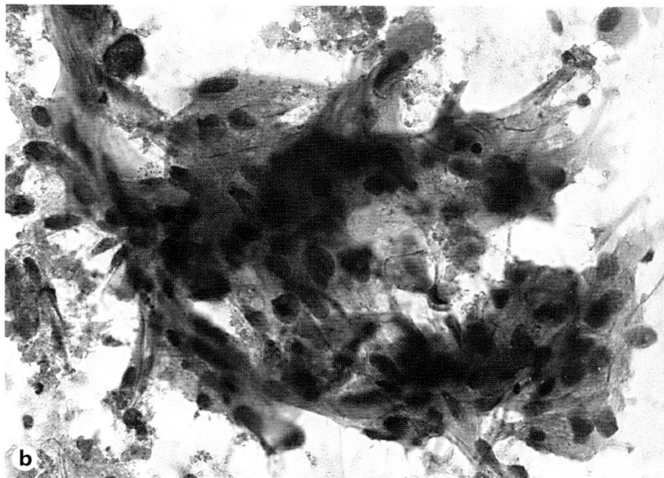

Fig. 29. Cytology of metaplastic carcinoma. The most frequent cytological aspects from metaplastic carcinomas include hypercellular clusters of severely atypical cancer cells with "squamoid" cytoplasm in a dirty, often necrotic background. Papanicolaou. **a** Low power. **b** High power.

bular carcinomas or even as benign proliferative lesions if only the well-differentiated glandular component is detected [Bataillon et al., 2014]. The finding of squamous cells in breast FNAC is highly suspicious of the presence of a metaplastic carcinoma. Nevertheless, the presence of a purely squamous cell neoplasm in the breast should raise the doubt of being a metastatic lesion, so other possible sites of origin should carefully be ruled out.

The presence of chondroid matrix in the background can pose a challenging differential diagnosis with pleomorphic adenoma, myxoid fibroadenoma, and mucinous lesions (mucinous carcinoma and mucocele-like lesions). The presence of high-grade adenocarcinoma cells is usually sufficient to remove the doubt that it might be a benign lesion. However, some cases show well-differentiated tumor cells, and a definite diagnosis might be difficult if not impossible based on morphology only [Tajima et al., 2015].

Giemsa staining can be helpful to distinguish the chondromyxoid matrix of metaplastic carcinoma from mucinous material based on its typical brightly pink color, different from the blue to magenta shade of mucus.

A differential diagnosis between spindle cell metaplastic carcinoma and malignant phyllodes tumor might be possible on FNAC if an epithelioid component is present in the smear. Actually, malignant phyllodes tumor is composed of high-grade stromal cells and a benign-looking epithelial component, consisting of cohesive staghorn clusters of ductal cells with overlapping myoepithelial cells. Conversely, metaplastic carcinomas usually display elements resembling a poorly differentiated ductal or squamous carcinoma.

Tumors displaying only spindle cells in the smear might be impossible to define without the aid of immunocytochemistry. Sometimes, a definite diagnosis of metaplastic carcinoma is possible only on the surgical specimen.

Summary

Key Cytological Features of Metaplastic Carcinoma

- Malignant squamous cells
- Pleomorphic spindle cells
- Chondromyxoid matrix
- Necrotic debris in the background

Common Pitfalls of FNA: Metaplastic Carcinoma

- Only glandular elements with mild atypia (from a low-grade adenosquamous carcinoma)
- Only adenocarcinoma cells
- Metastatic squamous cell carcinoma
- Only bland-looking spindle cells

Adenoid Cystic Carcinoma

Introduction/Epidemiology

Adenoid cystic carcinoma of the breast is a very rare variant of breast carcinoma sharing morphological features with its analogue in salivary glands. It is usually found in

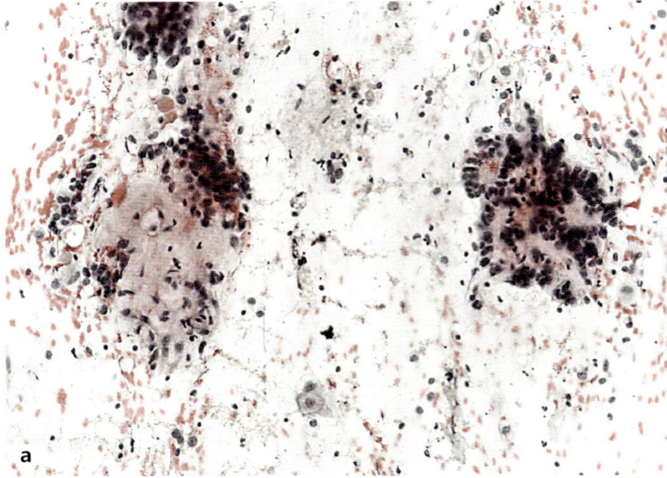

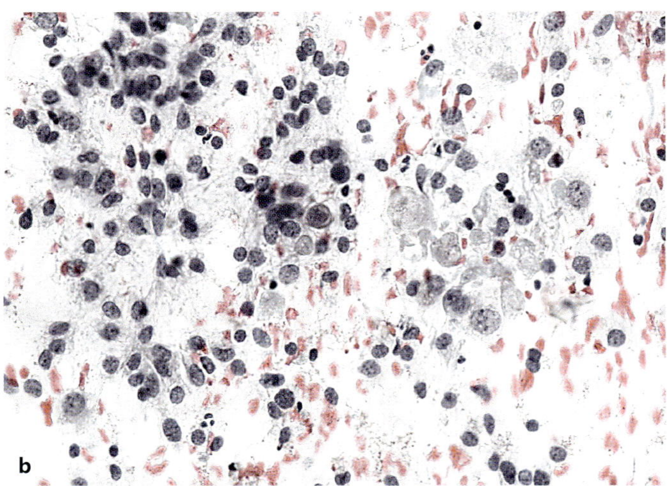

Fig. 30. Heterologous metaplastic carcinoma. Metaplastic carcinoma might be suspected on the cytological smear for the presence of chondromyxoid material in the background. Compare with Figure 28c (histology of the same case). The differential diagnosis is with myxoid fibroadenomas and mucinous carcinoma. Papanicolaou. **a** Intermediate power. **b** High power.

the sixth decade of life and seldom in premenopausal women. Tumor size may range from 0.7 to 10 cm, with an average of 3 cm in some series [Arpino et al., 2002; Peters and Wolf, 1983]. It fails to show the typical appearance of invasive ductal carcinoma on both mammogram and ultrasonography, usually presenting as a benign-appearing, smooth, round, or lobulated density or as an irregular mass (Fig. 31) [Sheen-Chen et al., 2005]. Symptoms at presentation include a breast lump and intermittent pain.

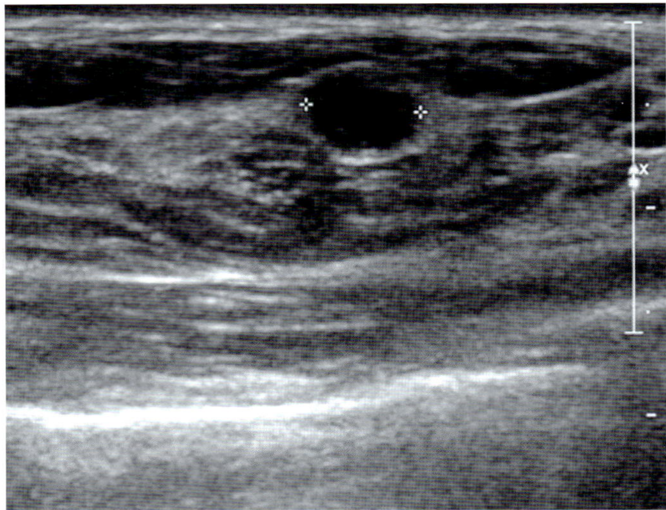

Fig. 31. Ultrasound of an adenoid-cystic carcinoma. This small lesion was initially considered benign based on radiological findings and turned out to be an adenoid-cystic carcinoma on the following cytological and pathological examination. On ultrasound, it appears as an ovoid, hypoechoic, partially cystic mass with round contours and the long axis parallel to the skin.

Histological Features

Similar to its analogue in salivary glands, adenoid cystic carcinoma of the breast is characterized by a variety of patterns that typically include small glandular lumina lined by ductal epithelium and eosinophilic "cylinders" with basement membrane material lined by basal/myoepithelial-type cells (Fig. 32). These tumors show an extremely low proliferative rate and have generally a good prognosis, with rare axillary lymph node involvement. Noteworthy, distant metastases might develop in a small number of cases, even though axillary lymph nodes are negative. For this reason, axillary lymph node dissection may not be helpful in this special type of cancer and probably should be avoided [Arpino et al., 2002].

ER and PR are variably positive, differently from adenoid cystic carcinomas of other sites, and Her2 is typically negative.

Cytology

The cytological appearance of adenoid cystic carcinoma reflects its peculiar histological aspect, showing clusters of epithelial cells oriented around solid spheres of amorphous, proteinaceous material. Cells are rather small and monotonous, with oval-shaped nuclei surrounded by a thin rim of

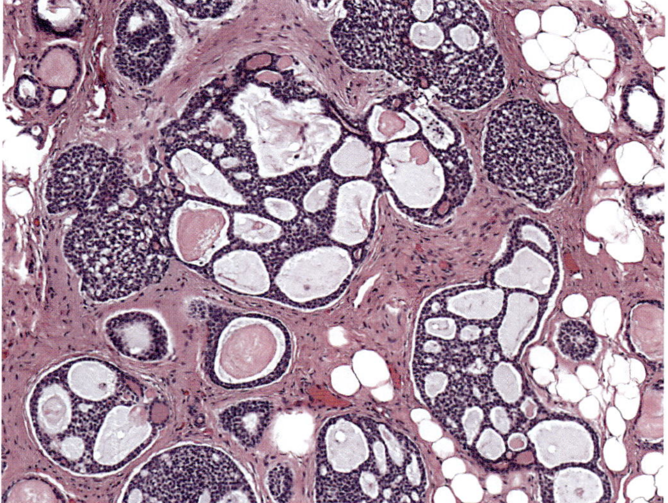

Fig. 32. Histology of adenoid-cystic carcinoma. The classical "cylindromatous" growth pattern is well represented in this case. Glandular lumina are filled with homogeneous, small, cuboidal cells lining variably sized cystic cavities with cylinders of eosinophilic material. H&E. Low power.

Fig. 33. Cytology of adenoid-cystic carcinoma. The typical picture of an aspirate from adenoid-cystic carcinoma includes small cellular clusters with round and neat borders composed of uniform cells with bland nuclei. Some clusters have small spheres of amorphous material in the center, around which display epithelial cells. Bare nuclei are present in the background, but they tend to be round rather than ovoid or bipolar. Papanicolaou. **a** Low power. **b** High power.

cytoplasm. Many bare nuclei are present in the background, but they tend to be round rather than oval or bipolar (Fig. 33).

The lack of cytological atypia, together with the radiological "benign" aspect, may lead to the misdiagnosis of this lesion as a benign proliferative lesion, such as microglandular adenosis or collagenous spherulosis. The latter is a peculiar condition rarely encountered in the breast, which shows collagenous spherules on cytological samples very similar to those found in adenoid cystic carcinomas. To differentiate both entities, attention should be paid to the nuclear/cytoplasmic ratio, which is very high in adenoid cystic carcinoma. Moreover, in collagen spherulosis, acellular spherules are surrounded by a single layer of cells, while in adenoid cystic carcinoma several layers may be present [Ilkay et al., 2015].

Besides the peculiar glandular aggregates with hyaline spherules in the center, a variable amount of tubular and solid clusters are often observed in aspirates from adenoid cystic carcinoma, and their presence, especially when numerous, may help in the differential diagnosis with other types of well-differentiated breast cancers. In these cases, the failed recognition of this entity may lead to a potential overtreatment of the patient, who would neither benefit from sentinel lymph node biopsy nor from axillary dissection. On the other side, the extreme rarity of this neoplasm should not lead the cytopathologist to a hurried, and potentially wrong, diagnosis. Thus, we suggest assessing aspirates suggestive of adenoid cystic carcinoma as "atypical or suspicious for carcinoma" and direct the patient to core needle biopsy to confirm the diagnosis before proceeding with the treatment.

Immunocytochemistry can be extremely useful to identify this neoplasm without resorting to core needle biopsy. Indeed, neoplastic cells are strongly positive for p63 and

CD117/c-kit, allowing a differential diagnosis with most invasive carcinomas (p63 negative) and collagenous spherulosis (CD117 negative) [Ilkay et al., 2015].

Summary

Key Cytological Features of Adenoid Cystic Carcinoma

- Moderate to marked cellularity
- Clusters of epithelial cells oriented around hyaline spherules
- Small-sized, bland cells with oval nuclei and scant cytoplasm

Common Pitfalls of FNA: Adenoid Cystic Carcinoma

- Tubular structures and solid aggregates
- Very mild cytological atypia
- Bare nuclei in the background
- Radiological "benign" aspect

References

Abdulla M, Hombal S, Al-Juwaiser A, Stankovic D, Ahmed M, Ajrawi T: Cellularity of lobular carcinoma and its relationship to false negative fine needle aspiration results. Acta Cytol 2000;44:625–632.

Arpino G, Bardou VJ, Clark GM, Elledge RM: Infiltrating lobular carcinoma of the breast: tumor characteristics and clinical outcome. Breast Cancer Res 2004;6:R149–R156.

Arpino G, Clark GM, Mohsin S, Bardou VJ, Elledge RM: Adenoid cystic carcinoma of the breast: molecular markers, treatment, and clinical outcome. Cancer 2002;94:2119–2127.

Bataillon G, Collet J, Voillemot N, Menet E, Vincent-Salomon A, Klijanienko J: Fine-needle aspiration of low-grade adenosquamous carcinomas of the breast: a report of three new cases. Acta Cytol 2014;58:427–431.

Blaichman J, Marcus JC, Alsaadi T, El-Khoury M, Meterissian S, Mesurolle B: Sonographic appearance of invasive ductal carcinoma of the breast according to histologic grade. Am J Roentgenol 2012; 199:W402–W408.

Bonzanini M, Gilioli E, Brancato B, Cristofori A, Bricolo D, Natale N, Valentini A, Dalla Palma P: The cytopathology of ductal carcinoma in situ of the breast. A detailed analysis of fine needle aspiration cytology of 58 cases compared with 101 invasive ductal carcinomas. Cytopathology 2001;12: 107–119.

Cyrta J, Andreiuolo F, Azoulay S, Balleyguier C, Bourgier C, Mazouni C, Mathieu MC, Delaloge S, Vielh P: Pure and mixed mucinous carcinoma of the breast: fine needle aspiration cytology findings and review of the literature. Cytopathology 2013; 24:377–384.

Dawson AE, Mulford DK: Benign versus malignant papillary neoplasms of the breast. Diagnostic clues in fine needle aspiration cytology. Acta Cytol 1994;38:23–28.

Di Saverio S, Gutierrez J, Avisar E: A retrospective review with long-term follow-up of 11,400 cases of pure mucinous breast carcinoma. Breast Cancer Res Treat 2008;111:541–547.

Eisinger F, Jacquemier J, Charpin C, Stoppa-Lyonnet D, Bressac-de Paillerets B, Peyrat JP, Longy M, Guinebretière JM, Sauvan R, Noguchi T, Birnbaum D, Sobol H: Mutations at BRCA1: the medullary breast carcinoma revisited. Cancer Res 1998;58:1588–1592.

Elston CW, Ellis IO: Pathologic prognostic factors in breast cancer. I. The value of histological grades in breast cancer. Experience from a large study with long-term follow-up. Histopathology 1991;19: 403–410.

Eusebi V, Magalhaes F, Azzopardi JG: Pleomorphic lobular carcinoma of the breast: an aggressive tumor showing apocrine differentiation. Hum Pathol 1992;23:655–662.

Ferlay J, Shin HR, Bray F, Forman D, Mathers C, Parkin DM (eds): GLOBOCAN v1.2, Cancer incidence and mortality worldwide: IARC CancerBase No. 10. Lyon, IARC, http://globocan.iarc.fr.

Fisher ER, Palekar AS, Redmond C, Barton B, Fisher B Pathologic findings from the National Surgical Adjuvant Breast Project (protocol No. 4) VI. Invasive papillary cancer. Am J Clin Pathol 1980;73:313–322.

Fu L, Tsuchiya S, Matsuyama I, Ishii K: Clinicopathologic features and incidence of invasive lobular carcinoma in Japanese women. Pathol Int 1998; 48:348–354.

Galzerano A, Rocco N, Accurso A, Ciancia G, Campanile AC, Caccavello F, Fulciniti F: Medullary breast carcinoma in an 18-year-old female: report on one case diagnosed on fine-needle cytology sample. Diagn Cytopathol 2014;42:445–448.

Gobbi H, Simpson JF, Borowsky A, Jensen RA, Page DL: Metaplastic breast tumours with a dominant fibromatosis-like phenotype have a high risk of local recurrence. Cancer 1999;85:2170–2182.

Helvie MA, Paramagul C, Oberman HA, Adler DD: Invasive lobular carcinoma. Imaging features and clinical detection. Invest Radiol 1993;28:202–207.

Hofmeyer S, Pekár G, Gere M, Tarján M, Hellberg D, Tot T: Comparison of the subgross distribution of the lesions in invasive ductal and lobular carcinomas of the breast: a large-format histology study. Int J Breast Cancer 2012;2012:436141.

Ilkay TM, Gozde K, Ozgur S, Dilaver D: Diagnosis of adenoid cystic carcinoma of the breast using fine-needle aspiration cytology: a case report and review of the literature. Diagn Cytopathol 2015;43: 722–726.

Jackman RJ, Rodriguez-Soto J: Breast microcalcifications: retrieval failure at prone stereotactic core and vacuum breast biopsy – frequency, causes and outcome. Radiology 2006;239:61–70.

Kashiwagi S, Onoda N, Asano Y, Noda S, Kawajiri H, Takashima T, et al: Clinical significance of the sub-classification of 71 cases mucinous breast carcinoma. Springerplus 2013;2:481.

Khandeparkar SG, Deshmukh SD, Bhayekar PD: A rare case of apocrine carcinoma of the breast: cytopathological and immunohistopathological study. J Cytol 2014;31:96–98.

Khurana KK, Wilbur D, Dawson AE: Fine needle aspiration of invasive micropapillary carcinoma of the breast. A report of two cases. Acta Cytol 1997;41: 1394–1398.

Lae M, Freneaux P, Sastre-Garau X, Chouchane O, Sigal-Zafrani B, Vincent-Salomon A: Secretory breast carcinoma with ETV6-NTRK3 fusion gene belong to the basal-like carcinoma spectrum. Mod Pathol 2009;22:291–298.

Lakhani SR, Ellis IO, Schnitt SJ, Tan PH, van de Vijver MJ: World Health Organization classification of tumours of the breast; in World Health Organization Classification of Tumours. Lyon, IARC, 2012, vol 4.

Lale S, Kure K, Lingamfelter D: Challenges to diagnose metaplastic carcinoma of the breast through cytologic methods: an eight-case series. Diagn Pathol 2011;6:7.

Menet E, Becette V, Briffod M: Cytologic diagnosis of lobular carcinoma of the breast. Cancer Cytopathol 2007;114:111–117.

Ohashi R, Sakatani T, Matsubara M, Watarai Y, Yangihara K, Yamashita K, Tsuchiya S, Takei H, Naito Z: Mucinous carcinoma of the breast: a comparative study on cytohistological findings associated with neuroendocrine differentiation. Cytopathology 2016;27:193–200.

Pai K, Baliga P, Shrestha BL: E-cadherin expression: a diagnostic utility for differentiating breast carcinomas with ductal and lobular morphologies. J Clin Diagn Res 2013;7:840–844.

Papadatos G, Rangan AM, Psarianos T, Ung O, Taylor R, Boyages J: Probability of axillary nodal involvement in patients with tubular carcinoma of the breast. Br J Surg 2001;88:860–864.

Pareja F, Corben AD, Brennan SB, Murray MP, Bowser ZL, Jakate K, Sebastiano C, Morrow M, Morris EA, Brogi E: Breast intraductal papillomas without atypia in radiologic-pathologic concordant core-needle biopsies: rate of upgrade to carcinoma at excision. Cancer 2016;122:2819–2827.

Patnick J (ed): NHS Breast Screening Programme. Annual Review 2010. Overcoming Barriers. Sheffield, NHS Cancer Screening Programmes, 2010.

Pedersen L, Zedeler K, Holck S, Schiodt T, Mouridsen HT: Medullary carcinoma of the breast. Prevalence and prognostic importance of classical risk factors in breast cancer. Eur J Cancer 1995;31: 2289–2295.

Peters GN, Wolff M: Adenoid cystic carcinoma of the breast. Report of 11 new cases: review of the literature and discussion of biological behavior. Cancer 1983;52:680–686.

Prathiba D, Rao S, Kshitija K, Joseph LD: Papillary lesions of breast – an introspect of cytomorphological features. J Cytol 2010;27:12–15.

Ranade A, Batra R, Sandhu G, Chitale RA, Balderacchi J: Clinicopathological evaluation of 100 cases of mucinous carcinoma of breast with emphasis on axillary staging and special reference to a micropapillary pattern. J Clin Pathol 2010;63:1043–1047.

Reid-Nicholson MD, Tong G, Cangiarella JF, Moreira AL: Cytomorphologic features of papillary lesions of the male breast: a study of 11 cases. Cancer 2006;108:222–230.

Reis-Filho JS, Milanezi F, Carvalho S, Simpson PT, Steele D, Savage K, Labmros MB, Pereira EM, Nesland JM, Lakhani SR, Schmitt FC: Metaplastic breast carcinomas express EGFR, but not HER2, gene amplification and overexpression: immunohistochemical and chromogenic in situ hybridization analysis. Breast Cancer Res 2005;7:R1028–R1035.

Robinson IA, McKee G, Jackson PA, Cook MG, Kissin MW: Lobular carcinoma of the breast: cytological features supporting the diagnosis of lobular cancer. Diagn Cytopathol 1995;13:196–201.

Robinson IA, McKee G, Nicholson A, D'Arcy J, Jackson PA, Cook MG, Kissin MW: Prognostic value of cytological grading of fine-needle aspirates from breast carcinomas. Lancet 1994;343:947–949.

Rosen PP, Cranor ML: Secretory carcinoma of the breast. Arch Pathol Lab Med 1991;115:141–144.

Sheen-Chen SM, Eng HL, Chen WJ, Cheng YF, Ko SF: Adenoid cystic carcinoma of the breast: truly uncommon or easily overlooked? Anticancer Res 2005;25:455–458.

Sheppard DG, Whitman GH, Huynh PT, Sahin AA, Fornage BD, Stelling CB: Tubular carcinoma of the breast: mammographic and sonographic features. Am J Roentgenol 2000;174:253–257.

Simsir A, Gomez-Aracil V, Mayayo E, Arraiza A: Papillary neoplasms of the breast: clues in fine needle aspiration cytology. Cytopathology 2002;13:22–30.

Simsir A, Waisman J, Thorner K, Cangiarella J: Mammary lesions diagnosed as "papillary" by aspiration biopsy: 70 cases with follow-up. Cancer 2003; 99:156–165.

Stalsberg H, Thomas DB: Age distribution of histologic types of breast carcinoma. Int J Cancer 1993;53: 1–7.

Tajima S, Koda K, Ishii Y, Hasegawa S, Yokoyama H: A case of matrix-producing metaplastic carcinoma of the breast exhibiting similarities to pleomorphic adenoma on fine-needle aspiration cytology. Int J Clin Exp Pathol 2015;8:15333–15337.

Toikkanen S, Eerola E, Ekfors TO: Pure and mixed mucinous breast carcinomas: DNA stemline and prognosis. J Clin Pathol 1988;41:300–303.

Toikkanen S, Pylkkänen L, Joensuu H: Invasive lobular carcinoma of the breast has better short- and long-term survival than invasive ductal carcinoma. Br J Cancer 1997;76:1234–1240.

Tse GM, Ma TK, Chu WC: Neuroendocrine differentiation in pure type mammary mucinous carcinoma is associated with favorable histologic and immunohistochemical parameters. Mod Pathol 2004;17:568–572.

Tse GM, Tan PH, Putti TC, Lui PC, Chaiwun B, Law BK: Metaplastic carcinoma of the breast: a clinicopathological review. J Clin Pathol 2006;59:1079–1083.

Tsuchiya S: Cytological characteristics of invasive lobular carcinoma of the human breast. Med Mol Morphol 2008;41:121–125.

Van Hoeven KH, Druids T, Cranor ML, Erlandson RA, Rosen PP: Low-grade adenosquamous carcinoma of the breast. A clinicopathologic study of 32 cases with ultrastructural analysis. Am J Surg Pathol 1993;17:248–258.

Ventura K, Cangiarella J, Lee I, Moreira A, Waisman J, Simsir A: Aspiration biopsy of mammary lesions with abundant extracellular mucinous material. Review of 43 cases with surgical follow-up. Am J Clin Pathol 2003;120:194–202.

Vesoulis Z, Kashkari S: Fine needle aspiration of secretory breast carcinoma resembling lactational changes. A case report. Acta Cytol 1998;42:1032–1036.

Walford N, ten Velden J: Histiocytoid breast carcinoma: an apocrine variant of lobular carcinoma. Histopathology 1989;14:515–522.

Walsh MM, Bleiweiss IJ: Invasive micropapillary carcinoma of the breast: 80 cases of an underrecognized entity. Hum Pathol 2001;32:583–589.

Zhang L, Jia N, Han L, Yang L, Xu W, Chen W: Comparative analysis of imaging and pathology features of mucinous carcinoma of the breast. Clin Breast Cancer 2015;15:147–154.

Pinamonti M, Zanconati F: Breast Cytopathology. Assessing the Value of FNAC in the Diagnosis of Breast Lesions.
Monogr Clin Cytol. Basel, Karger, 2018, vol 24, pp 94–99 (DOI: 10.1159/000479770)

Other Breast Neoplasms

Angiosarcoma

Introduction/Epidemiology

Angiosarcomas of the breast are relatively rare, but they represent the second most common mesenchymal malignancy in the breast after high-grade phyllodes tumor. They are classically subdivided into primary and secondary angiosarcomas based on their clinical presentation. Primary angiosarcomas are rare and may occur in younger women, usually in the third or fourth decade of life. They develop deeply in the breast parenchyma as painless masses or diffuse breast enlargement. Secondary angiosarcomas arise in the breast skin or in the chest wall in patients who underwent breast surgery, as a consequence of lymphedema after axillary dissection or, most commonly nowadays, after conservative breast surgery (lumpectomy or quadrantectomy for breast carcinoma) followed by radiation treatment [Mery et al., 2009]. These lesions are frequently multifocal and may be preceded by atypical vascular proliferation in the breast skin, appearing as small, reddish intradermal nodules over the treated area.

The mammographic findings are nonspecific, generally showing ill-defined and noncalcified masses, while ultrasound, especially color Doppler sonography, might help to visualize hypervascularized lesions. Secondary angiosarcomas presenting as cutaneous plaques may be difficult to differentiate by ultrasound from the thickened dermis after radiation treatment [Glazebrook et al., 2008].

Histological Features

Low-grade angiosarcoma appears as a proliferation of anastomosing vascular channels that infiltrate the surrounding tissue. Neoplastic endothelial cells show prominent and hyperchromatic nuclei and may grow inside the vascular lumen forming pseudopapillary projections. Poorly differentiated angiosarcoma is easily recognized as a malignant neoplasm, but its vascular nature may be less evident. Irregular and anastomosing vascular channels are intermingled with solid cellular areas with spindle or epithelioid morphology; blood lakes, necrotic areas, and mitoses are typically present (Fig. 1).

Immunohistochemistry is usually required to confirm the diagnosis. Neoplastic cells express one or more endothelial markers (CD31, CD34, and D240/podoplanin) and are negative for cytokeratins.

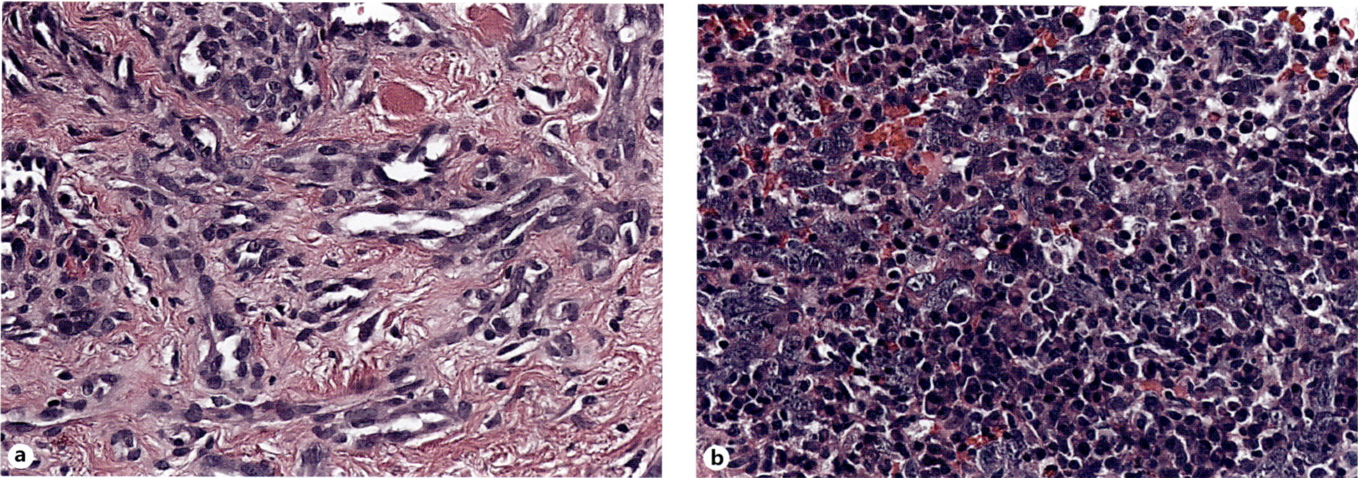

Fig. 1. Histology of breast angiosarcoma. Well-differentiated angiosarcoma shows proliferation of anastomosing vascular channels lined by endothelial cells with prominent nuclei (**a**). The vascular nature is harder to identify in high-grade angiosarcomas (**b**). H&E. Intermediate power.

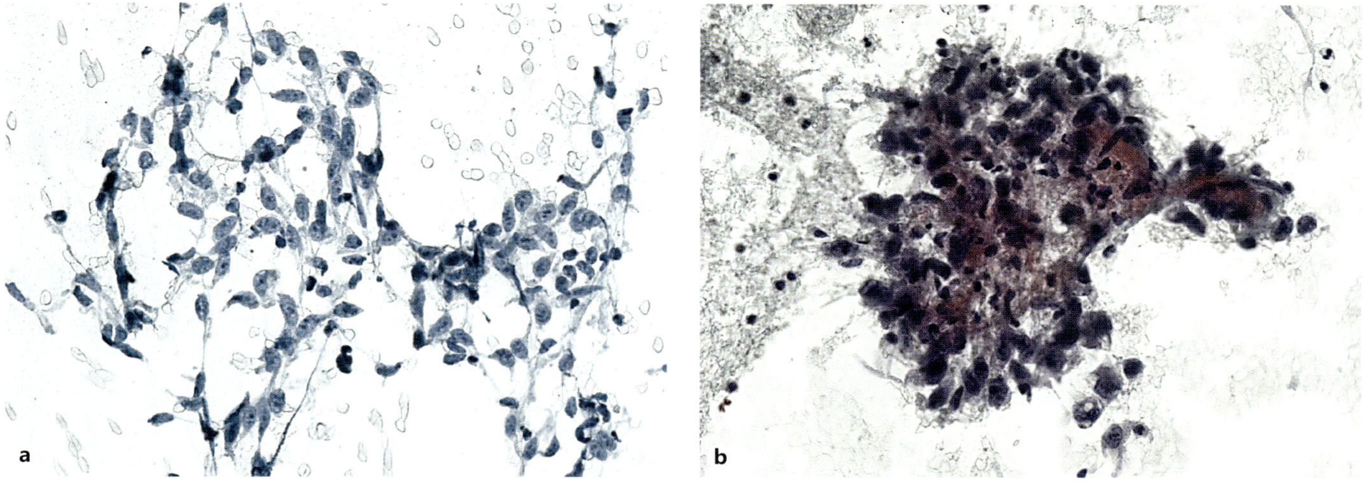

Fig. 2. Cytology of breast angiosarcoma. A population of spindle cells with plump nuclei and one or more nucleoli is a typical finding in aspirates from breast angiosarcomas (**a**). Nuclear pleomorphism, as well as cluster hypercellularity and debris in the background, is typically more evident in high-grade angiosarcomas (**b**). The background is frequently bloody in both low-grade and high-grade vascular neoplasms. Papanicolaou. High power.

Cytology

Aspirates from angiosarcomas are frequently bloody and contain a variable number of spindle and/or epithelial-like neoplastic cells showing nuclear atypia. Epithelial-like cells may be arranged in tight clusters with papillary configuration and resemble carcinoma cells. On the other hand, atypical spindle cells may raise the possibility of a fibromatosis-like lesion, a malignant phyllodes tumor, or a metaplastic carcinoma (Fig. 2). An accurate differential diagnosis is extremely difficult and sometimes impossible relying exclusively on morphology, and immunocytochemistry is necessary to verify the endothelial nature of the neoplastic cells [Markidou et al., 2010]. Clues that can help orienting the diagnosis towards an angiosarcoma include a bloody back-

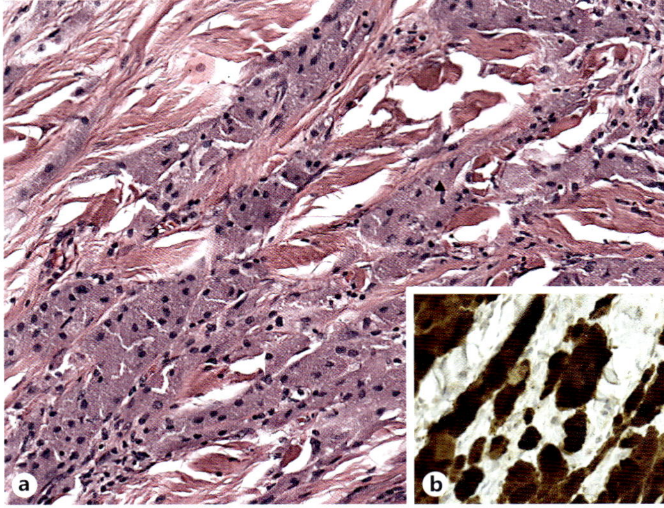

Fig. 3. Histology of granular cell tumor. The lesion is composed of a population of cells with small and bland nuclei and wide granular and eosinophilic cytoplasm dissecting the collagen bundles (**a**). Strong and diffuse S-100 positivity confirms the neuroid nature of the lesion (**b**). H&E (**a**) and S-100 immunohistochemistry (**b**). Intermediate power.

ground and clinical history of previous surgery and radiation [Chhieng et al., 1999]. We recommend performing skin biopsy or core needle biopsy in cases that are suspicious for angiosarcoma.

Granular Cell Tumor

Introduction/Epidemiology

Also known as Abrikossoff tumor, the granular cell tumor is an uncommon neoplasm derived from Schwann cells of peripheral nerves that can occur in the breast as well as many different organs. It is almost always benign [Lack et al., 1980] but may mimic malignancy on both radiological and clinical presentation. It usually appears as a single, 1- to 5-cm, irregular, firm mass in the breast parenchyma, may cause skin retraction, nipple inversion, or involve pectoralis fascia. Moreover, it has been found in association with mastectomy scars and might erroneously be interpreted as a recurrence of the resected carcinoma.

Histological Features

The neoplasm is composed of cells with large, granular eosinophilic cytoplasm, arranged in sheets, clusters, or cords, with an infiltrative growth pattern. Nuclei are small, round to oval and uniform, displaying single evident nucleoli; mitoses are rare (Fig. 3). Malignancy might be suspected in tumors larger than 5 cm, with nuclear pleomorphism, increased mitotic activity, and necrotic areas. Attesting their neural nature, neoplastic cells are strongly positive for S-100 protein. The proliferative index is low (<20%).

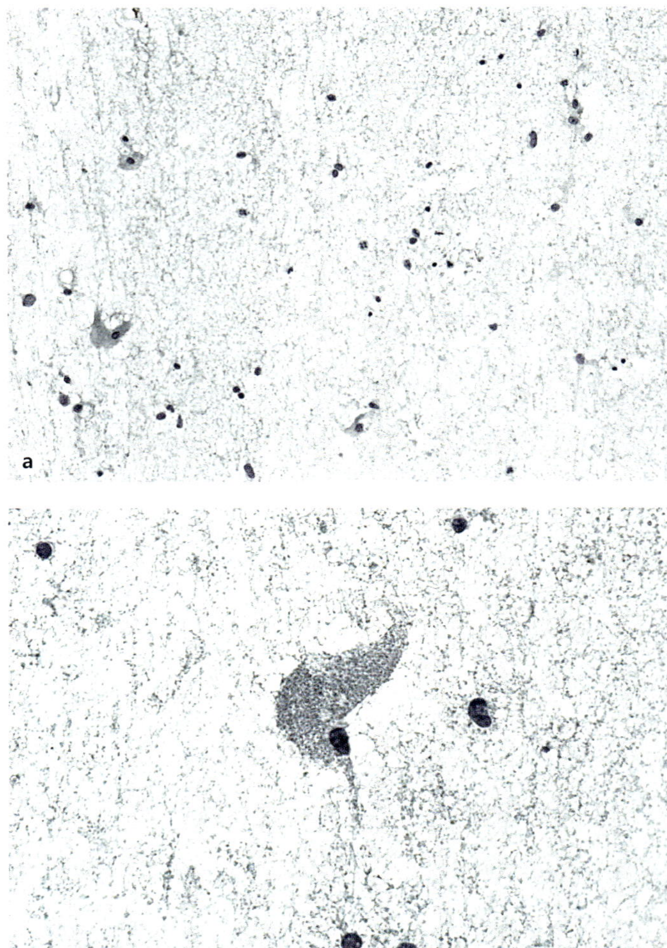

Fig. 4. Cytology of granular cell tumor. Aspirates from granular cell tumors are poorly cellular and show scattered dissociated cells with a small oval nucleus and wide granular cytoplasm, resembling histiocytes. Papanicolaou. **a** Low power. **b** High power.

Cytology

Aspirates are usually poorly cellular and show scattered dissociated cells with wide, granular cytoplasm and bland nuclei (Fig. 4). A differential diagnosis should be made with

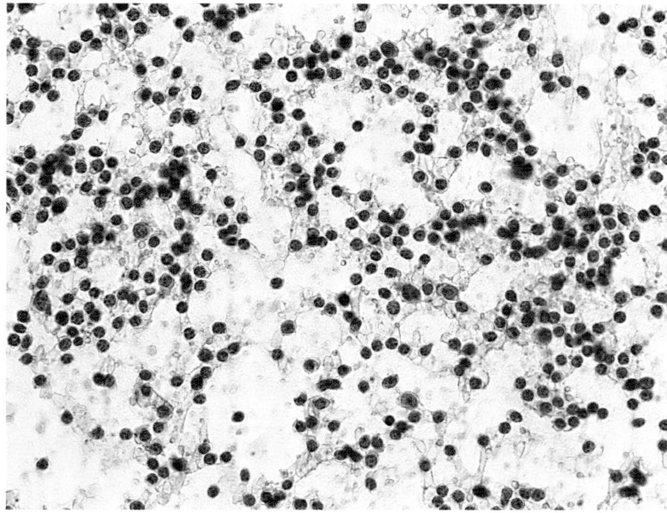

Fig. 5. Low-grade lymphoma (MALT lymphoma). The aspirate is dominated by a monotonous population of small lymphocytes with very mild atypia. The distinction from reactive lymphocytic proliferation is extremely difficult if not impossible based on morphology alone and usually relies on ancillary tests or histology. Papanicolaou. High power.

apocrine lesions and histiocytic proliferations. Importantly, cells should be distinguished from those of an apocrine carcinoma, which may result in unnecessary treatment following misdiagnosis. Careful examination of the nuclei is the key diagnostic element to rule out a carcinoma, while the cytoplasm, which is granular rather than foamy, could allow the distinction from histiocytes. Immunocytochemistry could be useful to confirm the diagnosis.

When correctly recognized, this lesion should be assessed as benign. Also, this result is in most cases a source of discrepancy with the clinical and radiological findings, and a diagnostic biopsy is frequently required.

Lymphomas

Non-Hodgkin's lymphomas represent the most common nonepithelial tumors of the breast. Lymphomas may arise primarily in the breast or involve it as a consequence of their diffusion throughout the body [Arora et al., 2013]. B-cell neoplasms are far more common than T-cell neoplasms; diffuse large B-cell lymphomas (DLBCL) are most often encountered, accounting for 53% of all primary breast lymphomas. Other uncommon types include the Burkitt lymphoma, MALT lymphoma, and follicular lymphoma [Domchek et al., 2002]. Like other extranodal lymphomas, these are more common in human immunodeficiency virus-infected patients and may represent the first manifestation of the disease.

The clinical and radiological features of breast lymphomas are usually suspicious for the presence of a carcinoma. On the mammogram, they typically appear as relatively circumscribed opacities that usually do not contain any calcification [Liberman et al., 1994].

Aspirates from breast lymphomas usually show a disperse population of variably atypical lymphoid cells, which can be larger or smaller depending on the type and grade of the lymphoma. DLBCLs usually display a monomorphic population of relatively large cells that are 2–3 times larger than normal mature lymphocytes and show enlarged rounded nuclei, fine granular chromatin, and prominent nucleoli. The distinction from an epithelial neoplasia is based mainly on the grade of cellular dissociation together with the extremely high nuclear/cytoplasmic ratio. Still, it can simulate a lobular carcinoma or a metastatic small cell carcinoma, but features such as cytoplasmic vacuolization, single cells, and nuclear molding are generally absent. A medullary breast carcinoma might enter the differential diagnosis, but in DLBCL a single population of atypical cells is usually present rather than the bimodal pattern of neoplastic epithelial cells and reactive polymorphic infiltrate. In selected cases, immunocytochemistry for CD45 and cytokeratins might be helpful.

Low-grade lymphomas usually display a monotonous population of small lymphocytes with slight nuclear abnormalities; in such cases, the diagnosis of a lymphoma can only be suspected based on morphology alone, since a sure distinction from a reactive process or an intraparenchymal lymph node cannot be made (Fig. 5). Absence of macrophages with tingible bodies [see Chapter 10, this vol., pp. 100–105] and the extreme monotony of the lymphocytic cell population are clues that may direct the diagnosis towards a low-grade lymphoma. Immunocytochemical staining for CD3 and CD20, as a first approach, can evidence an imbalance in the ratio between B and T cells, supporting the suspicion of a low-grade lymphoma.

Immunocytochemistry, whether on cell blocks or direct smears, cannot only support or confirm a diagnosis of lymphoma, in expert hands it can also be a useful tool for the characterization of the lymphoma, possibly guiding the therapeutic approach [Arora et al., 2013].

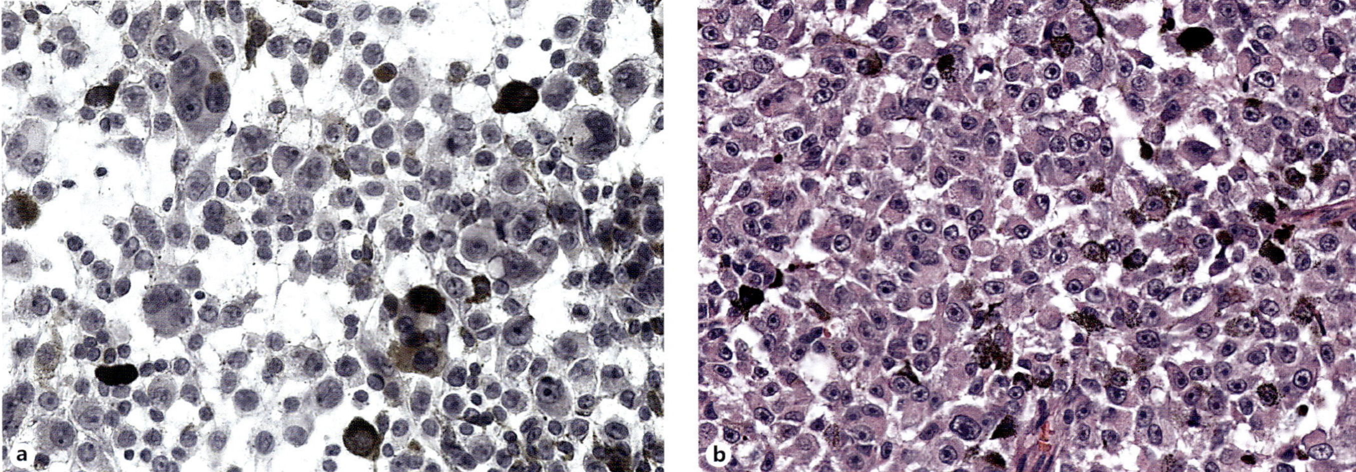

Fig. 6. Malignant melanoma. Neoplastic cells in the aspirate are mainly dissociated and display one or more large nuclei with prominent nucleoli. Melanin pigment is evident in the cytoplasm in this case (**a**). The same aspects are evident in the histological sample from the same lesion (**b**). Papanicolaou (**a**) and H&E (**b**). High power.

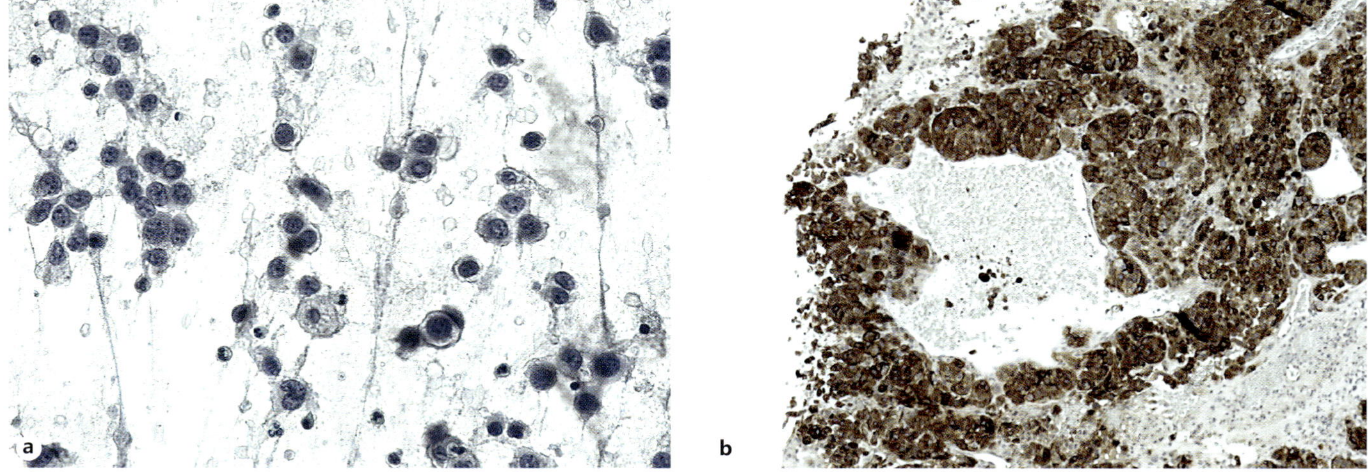

Fig. 7. Malignant melanoma, amelanic. Malignant melanoma is well known as a mimic of other neoplasms. This case, lacking the distinctive features of melanomas, such as melanin pigment and prominent nucleoli, was diagnosed as carcinoma on the aspirate (**a**). A diagnosis of malignant melanoma was made on the subsequent biopsy based on the results of immunohistochemistry (**b**). Papanicolaou (**a**) and Melan A immunohistochemistry (**b**). **a** High power. **b** Low power.

Metastases to the Breast

The breast is an uncommon site of metastases, but metastatic tumors exist and represent about 0.2–1.3% of all malignancies in the breast [Alvarado Cabrero et al., 2003]. In 30% of cases, the breast lesion is the first sign of the disease.

Tumors that most commonly metastasize to the breast include lymphomas, carcinomas – mainly from the lung, ovary, and skin – and malignant melanomas. The radiological findings are not significantly different from those of primary breast carcinomas, with the exception of microcalcifications, which are generally absent in metastatic tumors, since they do not have an intraductal component. Moreover, metastatic tumors are more frequently multiple and have well-defined and rounded rather than spiculated margins. Clinically, metastases grow rapidly.

The correct cytological, as well as histological, recognition of a metastatic tumor in the breast usually requires clinical information on a previous or contemporary tumor at another site, unless the neoplasm shows some peculiar aspects, such as melanin pigment in malignant melanomas or keratinization in squamous cell carcinomas [Lee, 2007].

Malignant melanoma is one of the most common neoplasms metastasizing to the breast. Primary malignant melanomas of the breast parenchyma are reported in the literature, but they are exceptionally rare, and careful exclusion of another possible site of origin must be done prior to assess this diagnosis [Kurul et al., 2005]. Aspirates from malignant melanomas are usually cellular, showing a population of mostly dissociated pleomorphic elements with large nuclei, single prominent nucleoli, and scattered intracytoplasmic pigment granules (Fig. 6). Actually, malignant melanomas may show a wide variety of morphological aspects, and melanin pigment can be absent, and thus the diagnosis is only possible combined with immunostaining (Fig. 7). Melanoma cells are typically positive for S-100 protein, human melanoma black-45 (HMB-45), and Melan-A.

Another peculiar neoplasm that can be diagnosed as a metastasis to the breast is small cell carcinoma of the lung. FNAC may allow a diagnosis of small cell carcinoma for the presence of many small-sized neoplastic elements with extremely high nuclear/cytoplasmic ratio occurring either singly or in tight clusters in a necrotic background. These cells usually show a fine salt-and-pepper chromatin without clearly visible nucleoli, and crush artifacts, as well as mitotic figures, are typically present. Primary small cell carcinoma of the breast exists, but is extremely rare [Shin et al., 2000], while a metastasis from a lung primary is a more common occurrence, unfortunately carrying a more dismal prognosis. The radiological finding of a mass in the lung is usually sufficient to solve the case, but immunocytochemistry can be helpful as well. Lung small cell carcinomas typically express TTF-1 and are negative for estrogen and progesterone receptors, while breast small cell carcinomas tend to show the opposite pattern [Liu et al., 2009].

The recognition of a breast mass as a metastasis from another site is essential to set the most appropriate treatment and to determine the prognosis. Generally, mastectomy does not improve patient prognosis, but resection of the mass with appropriate margins might be helpful for a better control of the disease. Likewise, sentinel lymph node biopsy is useless in metastatic patients. Usually, the breast is not the only metastatic site, and patients have widely disseminated disease, thus the prognosis is poor.

References

Alvarado Cabrero I, Carrera Alvarez M, Perez Montiel D, Tavassoli FA: Metastases to the breast. Eur J Surg Oncol 2003;29:854–855.

Arora SK, Gupta N, Srinivasan R, Das A, Nijhawan R, Rajwanshi A, Singh G: Non-Hodgkin's lymphoma presenting as breast masses: a series of 10 cases diagnosed on FNAC. Diagn Cytopathol 2013;41:53–59.

Chhieng DC, Cangiarella JF, Waisman J, Fernandez G, Cohen JM: Fine-needle aspiration cytology of spindle cell lesions of the breast. Cancer Cytopathol 1999;87:359–371.

Domchek SM, Hecht JL, Fleming MD, Pinkus GS, Canellos GP: Lymphomas of the breast – primary and secondary involvement. Cancer 2002;94:6–13.

Glazebrook KN, Magut MJ, Reynolds C: Angiosarcoma of the breast. AJR Am J Roentgenol 2008;190:533–538.

Kurul S, Tas F, Buyukbabani N, et al: Different manifestations of malignant melanoma in the breast: a report of 12 cases and a review of the literature. Jpn J Clin Oncol 2005;35:202–206.

Lack EE, Worsham GF, Callihan MD, Crawford BE, Klappenbach S, Rowden G, Chun B: Granular cell tumour: a clinicopathologic study of 110 patients. J Surg Oncol 1980;13;301–316.

Lee AH: The histological diagnosis of metastases to the breast from extramammary malignancies. J Clin Pathol 2007;60:1333–1341.

Liberman L, Giess CS, Dershaw DD, Louie DC, Deutch BM: Non-Hodgkin lymphoma of the breast: imaging characteristics and correlation with histopathologic findings. Radiology 1994;192:157–160.

Liu W, Palma-Diaz F, Alasio TM: Primary small cell carcinoma of the lung initially presenting as a breast mass: a fine-needle aspiration diagnosis. Diagn Cytopathol 2009;37:208–212.

Markidou S, Karydas I, Papadopoulos S, Christodoulidou I, Skarpidi E, Maounis N: Fine needle aspiration cytology in primary breast angiosarcoma: a case report. Acta Cytol 2010;54(5 suppl):764–770.

Mery CM, George S, Bertagnolli MM, Raut CP: Secondary sarcomas after radiotherapy for breast cancer: sustained risk and poor survival. Cancer 2009;115:4055–4063.

Shin SJ, Delellis RA, Ying L, Rosen PP: Small cell carcinoma of the breast: a clinicopathologic and immunohistochemical study of nine patients. Am J Surg Pathol 2000;24:1231–1238.

Pinamonti M, Zanconati F: Breast Cytopathology. Assessing the Value of FNAC in the Diagnosis of Breast Lesions.
Monogr Clin Cytol. Basel, Karger, 2018, vol 24, pp 100–105 (DOI: 10.1159/000479772)

Assessment of the Lymph Node Status

Lymph node status is the single most important prognostic factor in patients with breast carcinoma [Fitzgibbons et al., 2000]. Traditionally, it has been evaluated by routine axillary lymph node dissection performed concomitant with lumpectomy or mastectomy, but this practice has resulted in unnecessary mutilation and side effects, such as neuropathy and lymphedema, in a large number of patients with negative lymph nodes. The increased detection of lesions at an early stage based on mammographic screening fostered research on alternative methods to assess the lymph node status in patients with breast cancer.

Nowadays, the combined preoperative clinical, ultrasound, and FNAC approach, together with sentinel lymph node (SLN) biopsy, can avoid unnecessary dissection in most patients with negative lymph nodes, allowing also the early recognition of metastases prior to surgery.

Anatomical Basis of Breast Lymphatic Drainage

Lymphatic drainage of the breast is collected via the subareolar plexus and then follows three different routes. The majority of lymph (>75%), and especially that coming from the upper and outer quadrants, is drained through the axillary pathway, which runs around the inferior edge of the pectoralis major and reaches the pectoral group of axillary lymph nodes. Some of the lymph drained from both the medial and lateral part of the breast is drained through the internal mammary pathway, which passes through the pectoralis major and reaches the internal mammary lymph node chain. From this pathway, a small part of the lymph may reach the contralateral breast. The retromammary pathway collects the lymph coming from the posterior portion of the breast.

Hints of Radiological Findings in Lymph Nodes

Clinical examination of the axilla, which usually completes the clinical breast examination, may evidence suspicious palpable nodes, but its sensitivity and specificity are generally low. Ultrasound can easily explore the different lymph node chains and analyze the shape and echogenicity of the lymph nodes. A normal or reactive lymph node is small (usually up to 1 cm) and oval or bean shaped, and has a hyperechoic central part corresponding to the hilum and hypoechoic cortex. Metastatic disease is indicated by the 2-dimensional enlargement of the lymph node, which becomes round or sometimes irregular, in the absence of the echogenic hilum and irregularity or thickening of the cortex (Fig. 1) [Rizzatto, 2001]. In some cases, axillary lymph nodes might be visible already on the mammogram, especially if enlarged (Fig. 2).

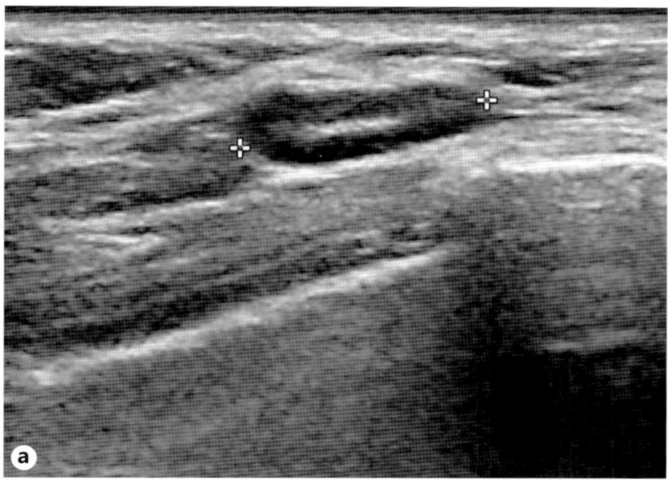

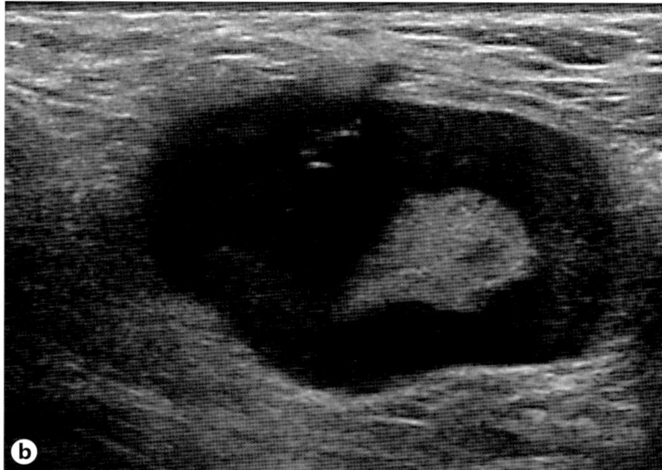

Fig. 1. Ultrasound imaging of axillary lymph nodes. A normal lymph node is typically oval- or bean-shaped and hypoechoic, with a hyperechoic hilar region (**a**). The 2-dimensional enlargement of the lymph node, with thickening of the hypoechoic cortex and eventually disappearance of the hilar echogenicity, is important for a suspicious finding (**b**).

According to the guidelines from the National Cancer Institute sponsored conference [1996], radiologically indeterminate (BI-RADS 3), suspicious (BI-RADS 4), or malignant (BI-RADS 5) lymph nodes identified by axillary ultrasound must be further examined through FNA or core biopsy in order to rule out or confirm the presence of metastases and select the patients to be submitted to SLN biopsy or axillary lymph node dissection [Sapino et al., 2003]. When more than 1 suspicious lymph node is detected, only the largest or the one easier to approach should undergo FNAC, but if it turns to be negative, further examinations should be performed.

FNAC of Lymph Nodes

FNAC of axillary lymph nodes is a simple procedure and can be performed in the same way as FNAC of breast lesions. Similarly, rapid on-site evaluation of the aspirated material is suggested in order to minimize the patients recall because of an inadequate cytology. It is a reliable diagnostic method that allows to identify metastases preoperatively with very high specificity avoiding unnecessary SLN biopsy in positive cases [Bonemma et al., 1997; Gipponi et al., 2016; Sapino et al., 2003].

Before assessing the presence or absence of metastatic elements, the cytopathologist should be aware of the cytological aspects of a normal or reactive lymph node. An adequate

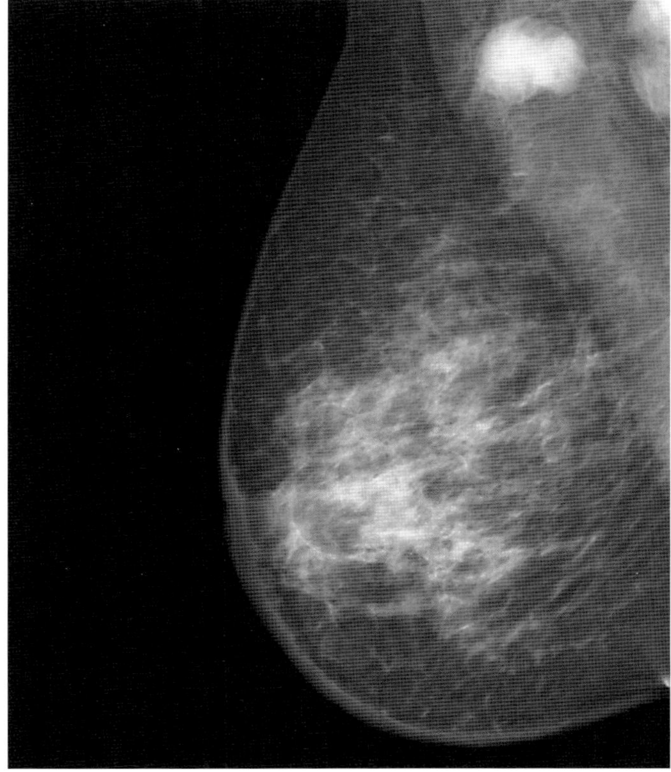

Fig. 2. Axillary lymph nodes on the mammogram. Enlarged axillary lymph nodes might be visible on the mammogram. In this case, a large, irregular opacity is visible in the axilla, corresponding to a metastatic lymph node.

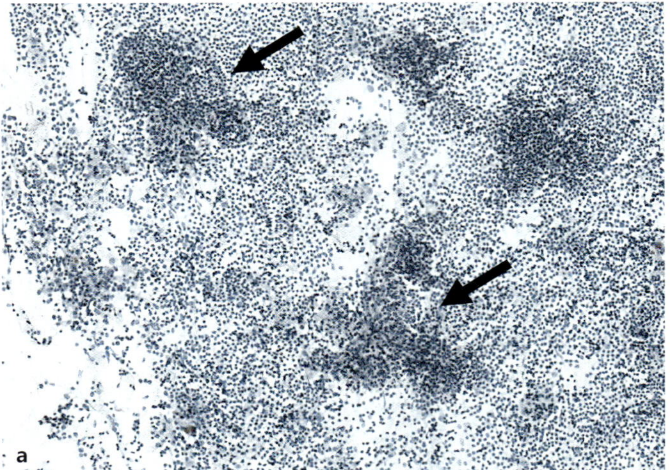

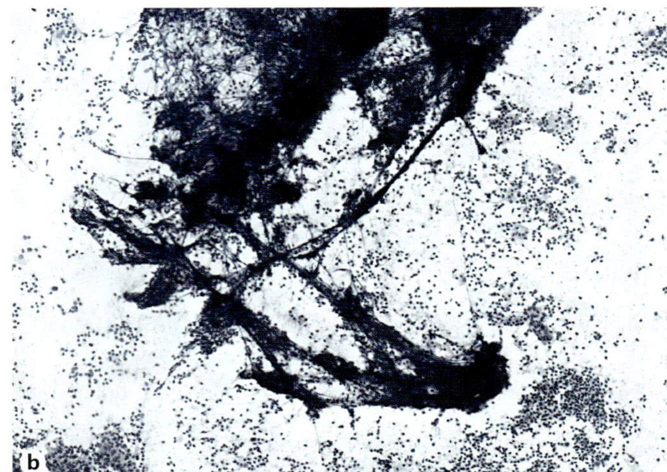

Fig. 3. Cytology of normal lymph nodes. Aspirates from axillary lymph nodes display a "carpet" of small lymphocytes admixed with other, less numerous, immune cells. Germinal centers are usually seen as poorly defined areas of densely packed cells (arrows) (**a**). Dark reticular structures composed of spindle-shaped cells and lymphocytes with crushed nuclei are a common finding in aspirates from lymph nodes (**b**). They are the result of the aspiration of sinusal histiocytes and vascular structures. Papanicolaou. Low power.

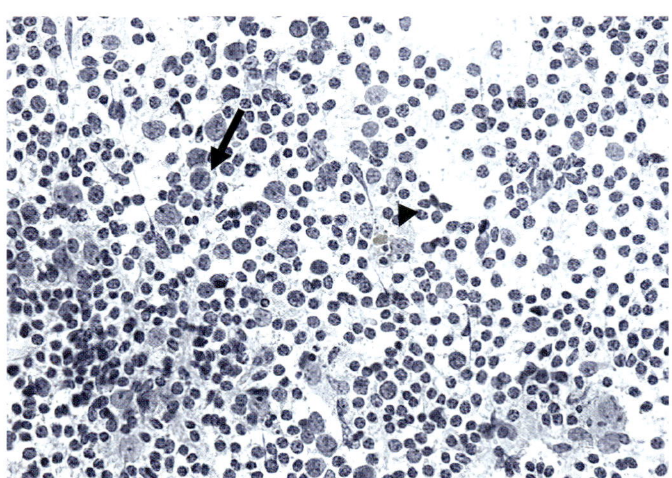

Fig. 4. Germinal centers. At higher magnification, germinal centers are composed of small lymphocytes, scattered larger lymphocytes with evident, "active" nucleolus (arrow), and epithelioid macrophages with abundant, pale cytoplasm, which sometimes contains cellular debris (tingible body macrophages) (arrowhead). Papanicolaou. High power.

aspirate from a normal axillary lymph node is moderately to highly cellular, displaying a polymorphous population of dispersed immune cells, among which lymphocytes predominate (Fig. 3). Lymphocytes are evident as uniform cells with nuclei that are a little larger than a red blood cell with a scanty rim of cytoplasm. The chromatin is dense, and nucleoli are not seen. Germinal centers are usually visible in the aspirate as loose aggregates of lymphocytes, follicular dendritic cells, and tingible body macrophages (Fig. 4). These macrophages have the function to phagocytose cellular debris of cells that undergo apoptosis in the center of the follicles and are an important sign of benign lymph nodes, since they are lost in some low-grade lymphomas that are otherwise very similar to normal lymph nodes, such as follicular lymphoma.

Other cells that are commonly encountered in reactive lymph nodes include mast cells, eosinophils, neutrophils, and sinus histiocytes. The latter can sometimes be loosely associated with each other simulating epithelial cells, not to be confused with cells of a metastatic tumor. The distinction can be safely made by careful examination of nuclear and cytoplasmic features.

Metastatic disease is easily detected when unequivocal carcinoma cells are present in the aspirate. This is the most common occurrence in clinically and radiologically suspect axillary lymph nodes in patients with a known breast carcinoma. Neoplastic cells are seen in such cases as a second "foreign" cell population that is strikingly different from the normal immune cells, show the typical epithelial cell-to-cell aggregation, eventually with 3-dimensional clusters, and have marked nuclear atypia (Fig. 5). Usually, theses cancer

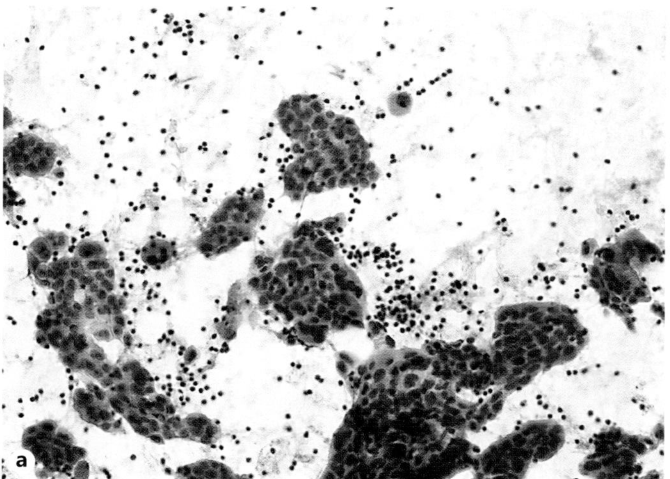
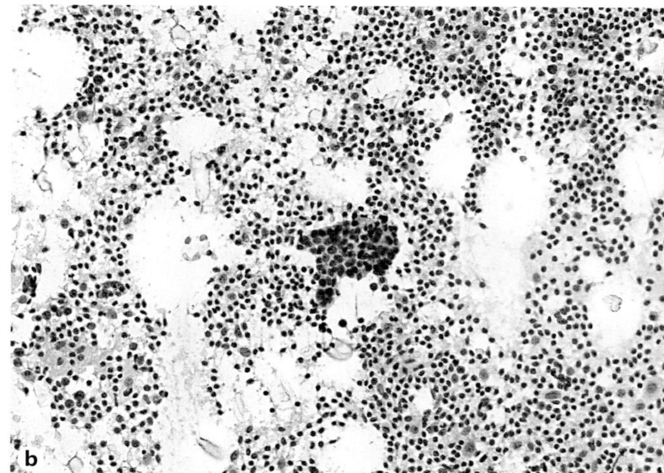

Fig. 5. Lymph node metastases. Metastatic cancer cells are evident in this lymph node aspirate and are well recognizable for the strong cell-to-cell adhesion and nuclear pleomorphism. The number of lymphocytes in the background may vary according to the portion of the lymph node occupied by the metastatic lesion (**a**, **b**). Papanicolaou. Intermediate power.

cells are present along with the lymphocytic population, but in the case of a massive metastasis with complete substitution of the lymph node parenchyma, lymphocytes might be scant or even absent. In such a situation, the term "lymph node metastasis" should be used carefully, because true lymph node cells are not detected in the smear, and the presence of a second cancer focus in a very peripheral site of the breast (or ectopic breast tissue) cannot be safely excluded.

Well-differentiated cancer cells do not show marked nuclear atypia but are generally arranged in cohesive groups and sometimes acinar or tubular structures, thus a distinction from immune cells is also relatively easy. Nevertheless, at least slight nuclear atypia should be appreciated before making a diagnosis of metastasis. Benign epithelial inclusions in axillary lymph nodes exist and are well documented [Kadowaki et al., 2007; Salehi et al., 2013], even if they are a very uncommon finding, and there are no reported cases of misdiagnoses in preoperative FNAC from axillary lymph nodes until now.

Lobular carcinoma represents a possible pitfall in cytological samples from axillary lymph nodes, since its cells are relatively small and lack cellular cohesion, simulating histiocytes, and it is the probable cause of many false-negative results, with the detection of cancer cells only in the definitive histological SLN examination. Lymph nodes that are highly suspicious by ultrasound but do not show striking abnormal cells at FNAC should be evaluated carefully in this view [Kim et al., 2016].

Sentinel Lymph Node Biopsy and Touch Imprint Cytology

SLN biopsy is now universally accepted as a valuable alternative to axillary dissection in patients with breast cancer and negative lymph nodes at preoperative examinations, and it is associated with significantly less morbidity [Krag et al., 2010]. Briefly, it consists of the selective excision of the first node(s) (usually 1–3) draining the lymph from a primary tumor, identified through the injection of a lymph tropic blue dye or radioactive tracer at the site of the neoplasm prior to surgery. These lymph nodes are then histologically examined and, if no metastases are found, the patient does not require axillary dissection, since the possibility of having lymph node metastases is about 1%.

There is still a wide variety in the methods used to perform the gross and histological evaluation of the SLN, whether cutting it in the long or short axis, with single or serial sectioning, and eventually the addition of immunohistochemistry to improve sensitivity [Apple, 2016; Ellis, 2005; Lyman et al., 2014]. Moreover, in many institutions, SLN undergo intraoperative examination, with the possibility of real-time identification of metastases. In such cases, the information passes directly to the surgical theater, where the patient undergoes axillary dissection without the need of a second intervention. The intraoperative examination can be performed on frozen-section analysis or imprint cytology [Cox et al., 2005; Pugliese et al., 2007] (Fig. 6). Most impor-

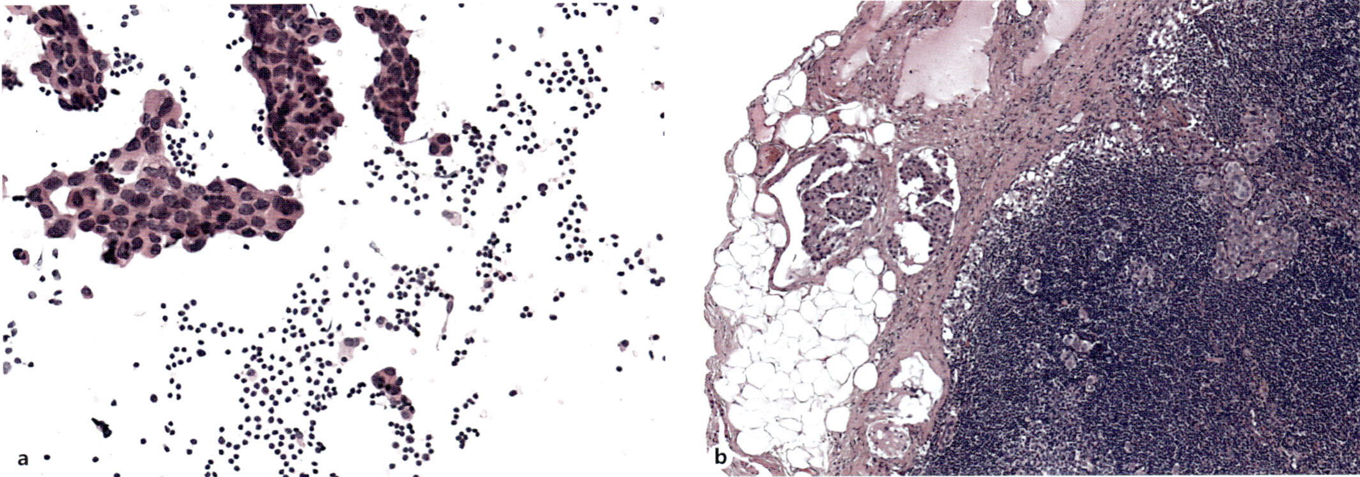

Fig. 6. Touch imprint cytology of axillary lymph nodes. Slides obtained through the touch imprint cytology may be fixed in 95% ethanol and rapidly stained with hematoxylin and eosin in the same way as histological frozen sections. Metastatic cells are evidenced by eosinophilic cytoplasm and the larger size of the nuclei compared to those of lymphocytes and macrophages (**a**). Touch imprint cytology does not alter the integrity of the tissue, which is then fixed in formalin and used for standard histological examination (**b**). H&E. **a** Intermediate power. **b** Low power.

tant for the purposes of cytopathology is the latter method, which has a proven efficacy in terms of both sensitivity and specificity and has the advantages of being less time consuming and of preserving the tissue quality for permanent sections [Sapino et al., 2003; Francz et al., 2011].

Performing imprint cytology is relatively easy, but some experience in cytopathology is required for a reliable microscopic evaluation of the samples. To obtain cytological smears from the lymph node, it must reach the laboratory fresh. Then, it is carefully separated from the adipose tissue and sectioned in 2- to 3-mm slices that are delicately and orderly arranged on a stable surface. A glass slide is superimposed on each lymph node slice and then gently spread by the use of another slide in the way shown in Chapter 1 [this vol., pp. 1–8]. Smears may be rapidly stained with Diff-Quick or Harris hematoxylin according to the cytopathologist's preferences and experience, and according to this decision should be air dried or immediately fixed in alcohol. Another method preferred by some cytopathologists is the scraping, by which the surface of the lymph node slice is gently scraped with a glass slide, which is then spread as usual. Finally, some authors combine the cytomorphological evaluation with rapid immunocytochemistry, eventually identifying cells of a metastatic lobular carcinoma, which could otherwise be missed by rapid evaluation [Sapino et al., 2003; Weinberg et al., 2004].

The way the smears are analyzed under the microscope is barely the same as FNAC from axillary lymph nodes, with the exception of the time the cytopathologist has available, which is much shorter. Most of the criticism that is moved against this practice is due to the relatively high frequency of doubtful or equivocal results compared to frozen sections. Dealing with intraoperative examination, whether histological or cytological, we believe that a potentially false-negative result is much less risky than an actual false-positive result, which not only burdens the patient with unnecessary treatments, but can also ruin the relationship of mutual trust between the surgeon and the pathologist, which is critical in view of today's close collaboration between different professionals. Atypical results are possible: they should be accompanied by a comment or explanation of the cytopathologist's doubts and perplexities, and should be interpreted as "negative" as regards the surgery in progress. Eventually, the axillary lymph node dissection could still be performed at a later time if metastases were identified on permanent sections.

Supporting this way of thinking is the recent trend of not performing axillary dissection in women with occult metastases and small breast tumors, who are treated with adjuvant hormonal therapy and/or chemotherapy in most cases [Maguire and Brogi, 2016].

References

Apple SK: Sentinel lymph node in breast cancer: review article from a pathologist's point of view. J Pathol Transl Med 2016;50:83–95.

Bonnema J, van Geel AN, van Ooijen B, Mali SP, Tjiam SL, Henzen-Logmans SC, Schmitz PI, Wiggers T: Ultrasound-guided aspiration biopsy for detection of nonpalpable axillary node metastases in breast cancer patients: new diagnostic method. World J Surg 1997;21:270–274.

Cox C, Centeno B, Dickson D, Clark J, Nicosia S, Dupont E, Greenberg H, Stowell N, White L, Patel J, Furman B, Cantor A, Hakam A, Ahmad N, Diaz N, King J: Accuracy of intraoperative imprint cytology for sentinel lymph node evaluation in the treatment of breast carcinoma. A 6-year study. Cancer 2005;105:13–20.

Ellis IO: Pathology reporting of breast disease. National Breast Screening Programme (NHSBSP) Publication. Publication No. 58. London, NHS Cancer Screening Programmes and The Royal College of Pathologists, 2005.

Fitzgibbons PL, Page DL, Weaver D, Thor AD, Allred DC, Clark GM, Ruby SG, O'Malley F, Simpson JF, Connolly JL, Hayes DF, Edge SB, Lichter A, Schnitt SJ: Prognostic factors in breast cancer. College of American Pathologists Consensus Statement 1999. Arch Pathol Lab Med 2000;124: 966–978.

Francz M, Egervari K, Szollosi Z: Intraoperative evaluation of sentinel lymph nodes in breast cancer: comparison of frozen sections, imprint cytology and immunocytochemistry. Cytopathology 2011; 22:36–42.

Gipponi M, Fregatti P, Garlaschi A, Murelli F, Margarino C, Depaoli F, Baccini P, Gallo M, Friedman D: Axillary ultrasound and fine-needle aspiration cytology in the preoperative staging of axillary node metastasis in breast cancer patients. Breast 2016;30:146–150.

Kadowaki M, Nagashima T, Sakata H, Sakakibara M, Sangai T, Nakamura R, Fujimoto H, Arai M, Onai Y, Nagai Y, Miyazawa Y, Miyazaki M: Ectopic breast tissue in axillary lymph node. Breast Cancer 2007;14:425–428.

Kim SY, Kim EK, Moon HJ, Yoon JH, Kim MJ: Is preoperative axillary staging with ultrasound and ultrasound-guided fine-needle aspiration reliable in invasive lobular carcinoma of the breast? Ultrasound Med Biol 2016;42:1263–1272.

Krag DN, Anderson SJ, Julian TB, Brown AM, Harlow SP, Costantino JP, Ashikaga T, Weaver DL, Mamounas EP, Jalovec LM, Frazier TG, Dirk Noyes R, Robidoux A, Scarth HM, Wolmarkl N: Sentinel-lymph-node resection compared with conventional axillary-lymph-node dissection in clinically node-negative patients with breast cancer: overall survival findings from the NSABP B-32 randomised phase 3 trial. Lancet Oncol 2010;11;927–933.

Lyman GH, Temin S, Edge SB, Newman LA, Turner RR, Weaver DL, Benson AB 3rd, Bosserman LD, Burstein HJ, Cody H 3rd, Hayman J, Perkins CL, Podoloff DA, Giuliano AE: Sentinel lymph node biopsy for patients with early-stage breast cancer: American Society of Clinical Oncology clinical practice guideline update. J Clin Oncol 2014;32; 1365–1383.

Maguire A, Brogi E: Sentinel lymph nodes for breast carcinoma: an update on current practice. Histopathology 2016;68:152–167.

National Cancer Institute sponsored conference. The uniform approach to breast fine-needle aspiration biopsy. Diagn Cytopathol 1997;16:295–311.

Pugliese MS, Tickman R, Wang NP, Atwood M, Beatty JD: The utility of intraoperative evaluation of sentinel lymph nodes in breast cancer. Ann Surg Oncol 2007;14:1024–1030.

Rizzatto GJ: Towards a more sophisticated use of breast ultrasound. Eur Radiol 2001;11:2425–2435.

Salehi AH, Omeroglu G, Kanber Y, Omeroglu A: Endosalpingiosis in axillary lymph nodes simulating metastatic breast carcinoma: a potential diagnostic pitfall. Int J Surg Pathol 2013;21:610–612.

Sapino A, Cassoni P, Zanon E, Fraire F, Croce S, Coluccia C, Donadio M, Bussolati G: Ultrasonographically-guided fine-needle aspiration of axillary lymph nodes: role in breast cancer management. Br J Cancer 2003;88:702–706.

Weinberg ES, Dickson D, White L, Ahmad N, Patel J, Hakam A, Nicosia S, Dupont E, Furman B, Centeno B, Cox C: Cytokeratin staining for intraoperative evaluation of sentinel lymph nodes in patients with invasive lobular carcinoma. Am J Surg 2004;188:419–422.

Pinamonti M, Zanconati F: Breast Cytopathology. Assessing the Value of FNAC in the Diagnosis of Breast Lesions.
Monogr Clin Cytol. Basel, Karger, 2018, vol 24, pp 106–112 (DOI: 10.1159/000479773)

Ancillary Techniques

Since Elwood V. Jensen's discovery in 1958 that estrogen receptors play a key role in the growth and survival of most breast cancers and the evidence that hormonal therapies could dramatically alter the history of patients, the diagnosis of cancer has been more and more associated with a series of additional information on prognostic and predictive factors. After that, between the 1990s and early 2000, a second sensational discovery brought another great change in the treatment and prognosis of breast cancer patients, since those with amplification of the human epithelial growth factor receptor 2 (HER2) gene, once burdened with a poor prognosis, could benefit from a targeted therapy, which sensibly improved their survival. Currently, the accurate assessment of the estrogen receptor (ER), progesterone receptor (PR), and HER2 status is essential and mandatory in all breast carcinomas [Allred, 2010].

If until 10 years ago molecular characterization could be performed directly on the surgical specimen, at present a change in the direction of patient management towards neoadjuvant therapies imposes more and more frequently a detailed characterization before surgical treatment, which is based on core biopsy or FNAC material [Hennigs et al., 2016].

The cytopathological methods available for this analysis are mainly immunocytochemistry (ICC) and in situ hybridization (ISH), which are briefly described in this chapter.

Immunocytochemistry

The presence and quantification of ER and PR in breast carcinoma cells can be evaluated using immunocytochemistry (ICC). Immunostaining can be performed on alcohol-fixed direct smears, like those used for Pap stains, as well as on liquid-based cytology (LBC) preparations and cell block sections.

Many laboratories with a long experience in cytology make large use of direct smears for immunocytochemistry, since it is possible to evaluate the adequacy of the sample, and specifically cancer cells can be found in the smear through morphological examination of the Pap-stained slide, which is then destained and used for ICC. However, direct smears may be problematic due to the presence of background material containing significant levels of cellular debris, especially in highly necrotic cancers, which may hinder a proper evaluation. Moreover, even more important, standardization of the ICC results is particularly difficult on direct smears. This is due to the differences in the protocols used for conventional cytology and the consequent differences in the quality of the cellular material.

LBC partly solves this problem thanks to its peculiar processing, and it can be very useful for ICC as well as molecular biology analyses [Rossi et al., 2010]. In contrast to direct smears, LBC enables to obtain many slides of comparable cellularity from a single sample, and this can be very useful when more than one staining is required, e.g., for prognostic and predictive markers in breast lesions. Like direct smears, LBC are pre-treated with an ethanol solution, and some antibodies may not be effective after such a treatment. ER results are not significantly affected by alcohol-based fixatives, while PR and HER2 staining has shown a variable concordance with the formalin-fixed slides [Hanley et al., 2009]. Moreover, all alcohol-fixed preparations usually need different concentrations (lower level) of the antibody in order to avoid false-positive results.

LBC serves not only as a method to support ancillary techniques, it might also be used for morphological diagnoses instead of direct smears, when the quality of conventional cytology is suboptimal, mainly due to bad spreading or fixation. On the other hand, the routine use of LBC in aspiration cytology might become problematic due to the inability to perform rapid on-site evaluation and the presence of different diagnostic criteria compared to conventional smears. For example, cells tend to lose their cohesiveness in a liquid medium, and background is frequently cleared out, potentially decreasing the diagnostic accuracy in certain lesion types [Mygdakos et al., 2009].

Cell block preparations are obtained by placing the aspirated material directly into a formalin-containing vial. It is then centrifuged, embedded in paraffin, and processed in the same way as histological material (Fig. 1). Several sections can be made, and thus several slides of comparable quality from a single sample can be subjected to multiple immunostaining methods. Moreover, since the material is treated in the same way as histology specimens, no special precaution has to be taken regarding the type and concentration of the antibody, and it is easy to compare the results with subsequent immunohistochemistry results of the surgical sample [Shidham and Falzon, 2010].

Similar to LBC, cell block cytology has the drawback of not being able to assess the adequacy of the sample during the aspiration session. Indeed, even if rapid on-site evaluation is performed on all conventional smears collected, the cell blocks still sometimes lack adequate cellularity for ICC testing. Ferguson et al. [2012] tested an original method that could overcome this problem by transferring cells from a direct smear to a gel medium, which was then embedded in paraffin and processed as cell blocks and standard histological material.

ER- and PR-stained slides are evaluated under the light microscope to determine the proportion and intensity of positive cells (Fig. 2). It is estimated that 80 and 60% of invasive breast carcinomas express nuclear ER and PR, respectively, in a proportion ranging from less than 1 to 100% positive cells. One percent is the established cutoff for ER and PR positivity by immunohistochemistry [Hammond et al., 2010]. ER and PR are strong predictors for the response to hormonal therapies such as tamoxifen [Early Breast Cancer Trialists Collaborative Group (EBCTCG), 2005]. This drug binds the receptor and blocks estrogen-stimulated growth and survival of tumor cells, with important consequences on the disease-free and overall survival of patients with hormone-sensitive tumors. The rate and intensity of the positive cells is correlated to the efficacy of the treatment, as it is the contemporary expression of ER and PR. The most frequent phenotype (70%) is ER+/PR+, which is associated with the best rate of treatment response (60%). ER–/PR– is the next most common combination (25%), and these tumors are essentially unresponsive. The remaining 2 discordant phenotypes are associated with intermediate response rates, although there is debate as to whether ER–/PR+ tumors actually exist [Lakhani et al., 2012].

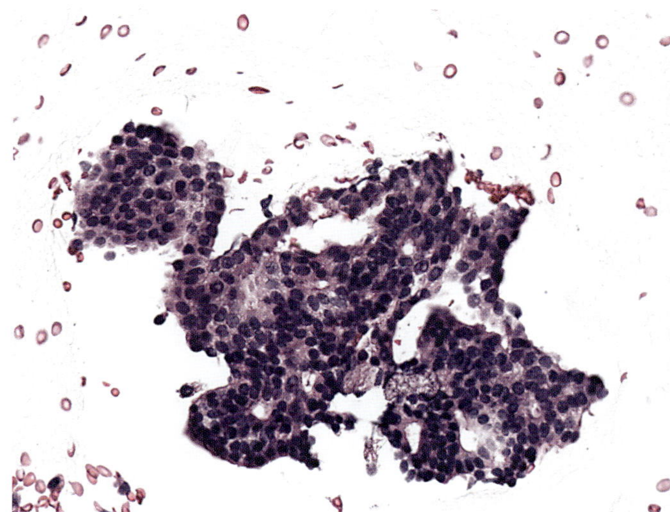

Fig. 1. Cell block cytology. This is a case of an invasive ductal carcinoma (no special type) that underwent FNAC. An additional pass was performed in order to obtain material for a cell block. Once adequacy was assessed based on the first H&E stain, further sections were used for immunostaining. H&E. Intermediate power.

The HER2 gene is amplified in approximately 15% of primary breast carcinomas, leading to elevated expression of the analogue protein on the cell membrane [Allred, 2010]. HER2-positive breast cancers respond favorably to drugs that specifically target the protein, such

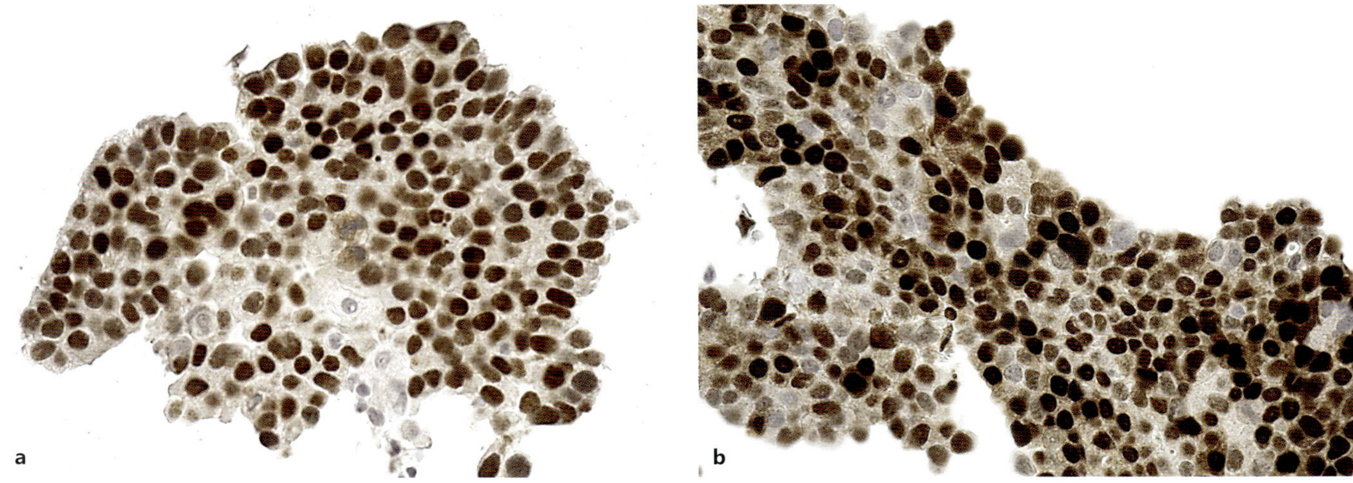

Fig. 2. Estrogen (ER) and progesterone receptor (PR) immunocytochemistry. This case shows diffuse and strong nuclear positivity for ER (**a**) and PR (**b**). Cell block immunocytochemistry. High power.

as trastuzumab, which on the other hand has a series of potential side effects and toxicity, and it should thus be administered only to patients who may benefit from the treatment.

The clearly HER2-positive cells may be easily identified by means of immunostaining for the presence of a strong circumferential membranous expression in most cancer cells (3+), although slighter positivity (2+) usually requires the use of in situ molecular techniques (Fig. 3). Complete absence of staining (0) or weak and incomplete immunostaining (1+) is considered a negative result. Guidelines have been developed to promote accurate testing for HER2 on formalin-fixed and paraffin-embedded tissue, but cytological samples are still lacking in such guidelines [Hammond et al., 2010; Wolff et al., 2007]. Concordance rates between HER2 immunostaining in alcohol- or formalin-fixed cell block preparations and histological samples are not optimal, with reported discrepancy rates of around 25% [Hanley et al., 2010; Kinsella et al., 2013].

There are many controversies in the use of cytological material for routine evaluation of prognostic and predictive markers of breast cancer. Controversies are not only limited to the variable performance of antibodies in alcohol-fixed samples, e.g., the frequent poor cellularity of cytological samples, the absence of internal positive controls, and the lack of standardization and universal guidelines for both the preanalytical and analytical phases. For these reasons, the routine analysis of these factors using FNAC should be limited to cases with no available tissue material, or otherwise a correlation with immunohistochemistry should be performed when possible [Kocjan et al., 2008].

Other markers that could be tested immunocytochemically to provide additional information to the cytological diagnosis include the proliferation of markers such as Ki-67, the adhesion protein E-cadherin, which can be useful to confirm or exclude a lobular carcinoma, the neuroendocrine markers chromogranin and synaptophysin, as well as other specific markers used to confirm or exclude the presence of a suspected metastatic neoplasm (e.g., Melan-A and CD45LCA) (Fig. 4–6).

Genetic Analyses

Molecular genetic techniques that are used in breast diagnostics include fluorescence ISH (FISH) or chromogen ISH and polymerase chain reaction (PCR). These techniques have proven to be suitable for FNAC as they do not require cell cultures and can be performed on relatively paucicellular samples. FISH has been traditionally used to assess the amplification status of the HER2 gene, especially in cases in which immunohistochemistry gives equivocal results. Cytology material obtained by FNAC has been shown to provide good quality of DNA with a yield that is comparable to that of core needle biopsy, and molecular in situ techniques performed on cytology material show an optimal concordance with histology [Symmans et al., 2003]. Furthermore, FNAC specimens generally contain even a greater rate of

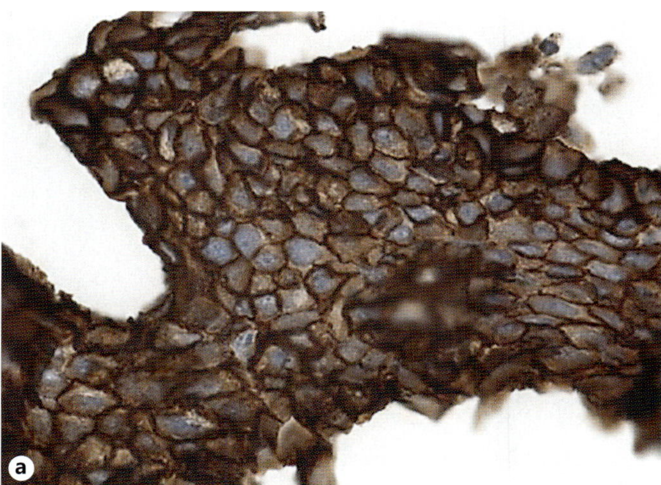

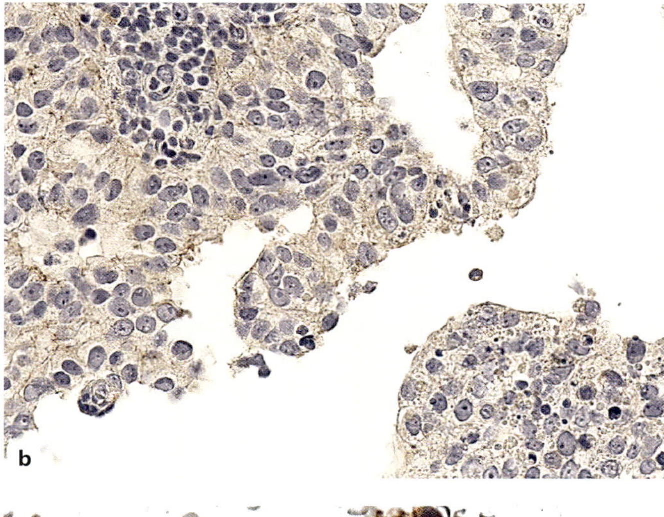

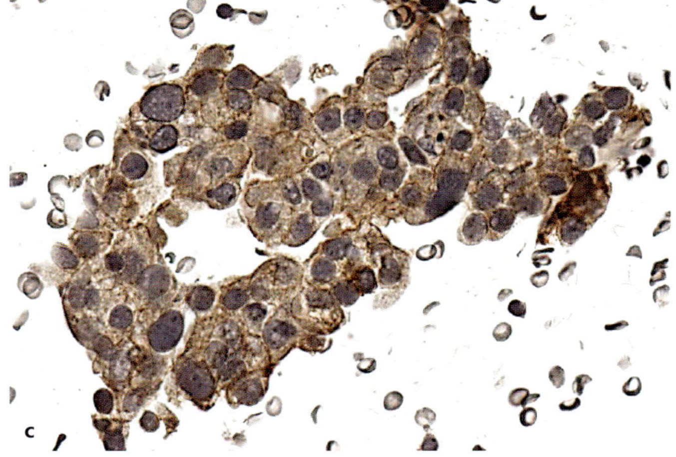

Fig. 3. HER2 immunocytochemistry. HER2 expression can be graded as 0, 1+, 2+, or 3+ based on the intensity and pattern of positivity. 3+ expression is defined as strong circumferential membrane staining in >30% of tumor cells (**a**). Cases with no staining or weak and partial membranous staining in <10% of tumor cells are considered completely negative (score 0) (**b**). Intermediate staining patterns are interpreted as equivocal (2+) and require further examination through in situ hybridization (**c**). Cell block immunocytochemistry. High power.

cancer cells than core needle biopsies, in which the stromal component is typically more represented and might in some cases result in contamination and lead to bias. Thus, FISH, as well as chromogen ISH, is an accurate technique for cytology [Beraki and Sauer, 2010]. PCR is another technique that has proven to be a reliable and fast method for the determination of HER2 status on cytological material aspirated from breast tumors [Rodriguez et al., 2016].

Molecular Classification of Breast Carcinoma

According to the expression of different gene combinations and proteins, breast carcinomas can be divided into several "molecular subtypes," not necessarily related to the classical histotypes listed in Chapter 8 [this vol., pp. 68–93], which are associated with different clinical outcomes and rates of response to treatment [Perou et al., 2000]. The so-called *luminal A* cancers express ER and PR, are HER2 negative, and have a low proliferative index (usually defined as Ki-67 <20%). *Luminal B* cancers have a similar molecular pattern but either lack the expression of one hormone receptor, express HER2, or have a higher proliferative rate. The other 2 molecular subtypes identified include *HER2-overexpressing* tumors, which are HER2 positive and hormonal receptor negative, and the so-called *triple negative* breast cancers, which neither express hormonal receptors nor HER2.

Luminal A tumors have generally a good prognosis and response to hormonal treatment, whereas luminal B cancers are more aggressive and more commonly require the use of chemotherapy and/or trastuzumab in addition to the hormonal treatment. HER2 overexpressing tumors behave in a very aggressive way, with rapid growth and early metastases, are unresponsive to hormonal treatment, but may show an

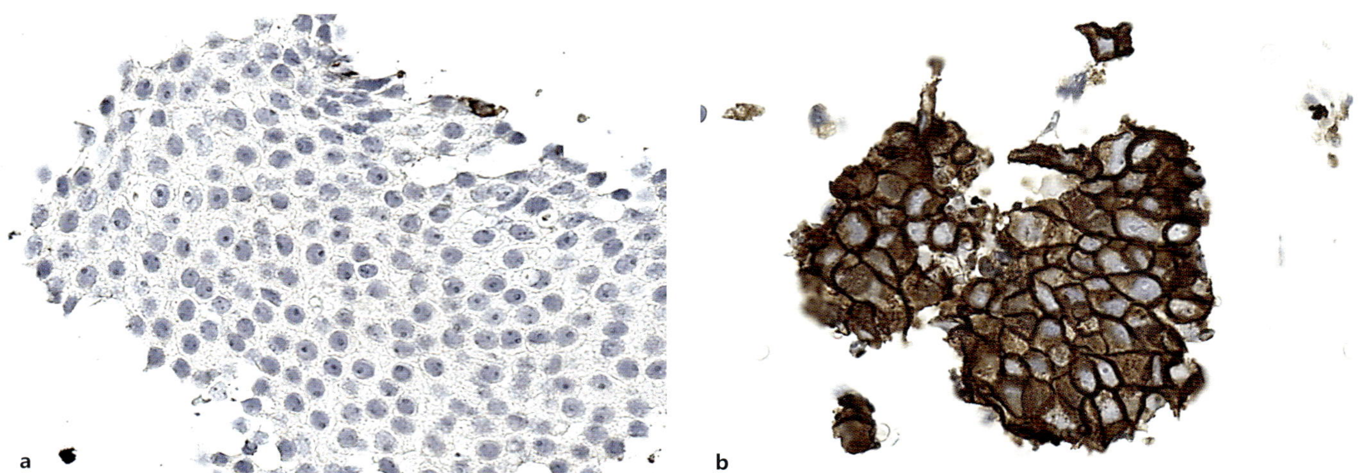

Fig. 4. E-cadherin immunocytochemistry. E-cadherin immunostaining can be used to differentiate lobular carcinoma, which is typically negative (**a**), from ductal carcinoma and other subtypes of breast cancer, most of which show strong and diffuse membranous expression (**b**). Cell block immunocytochemistry. High power.

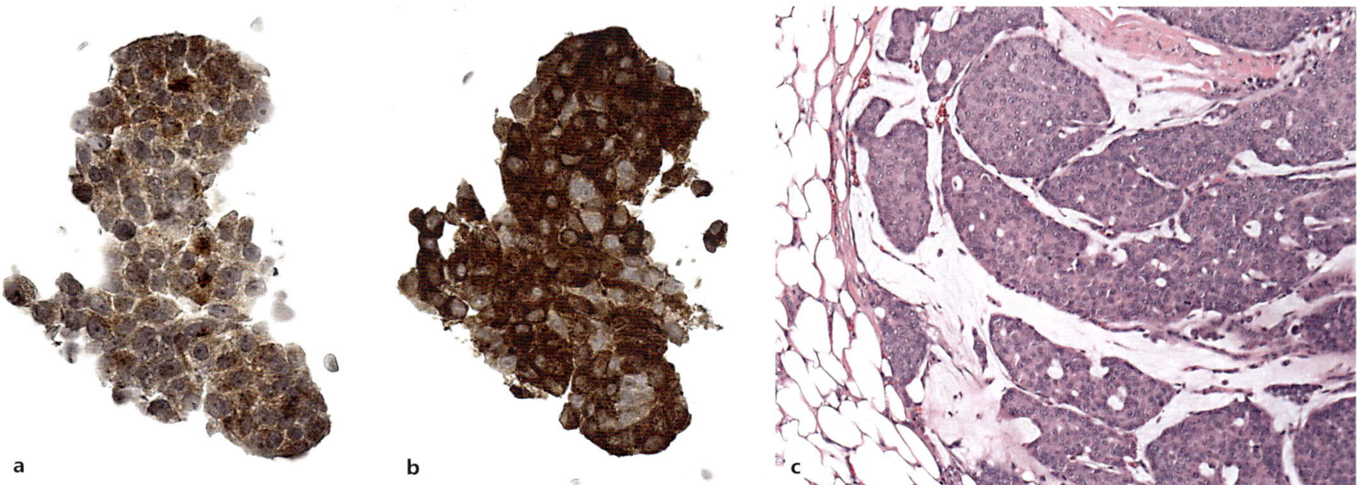

Fig. 5. Neuroendocrine markers. Chromogranin (**a**) and synaptophysin (**b**) immunostaining is commonly used to confirm the neuroendocrine nature of a neoplasm. Neuroendocrine differentiation can be found in many subtypes of breast cancer, but is more common in pure mucinous carcinomas (**c**). Cell block immunocytochemistry (**a**, **b**) and H&E (**b**). **a**, **b** High power. **c** Low power.

excellent response to targeted therapy. The triple-negative breast cancer category, comprising approximatively 20–25% of breast cancers, is a heterogeneous group including highly aggressive neoplasms, but also some relatively indolent tumors, such as most adenoid-cystic carcinomas and low-grade metaplastic carcinomas [Bauer et al., 2007; Geyer et al., 2017]. Basal-like breast cancers are included in the triple-negative category and are characterized by constitutive expression of genes usually found in normal basal/myoepithelial cells of the breast. They have generally a poor prognosis and are unresponsive to both hormonal and targeted therapies.

The distinction between molecular subtypes of breast cancer cannot be made on the basis of morphology alone. Although there are some morphological subtypes that frequently correspond to specific molecular types, such as

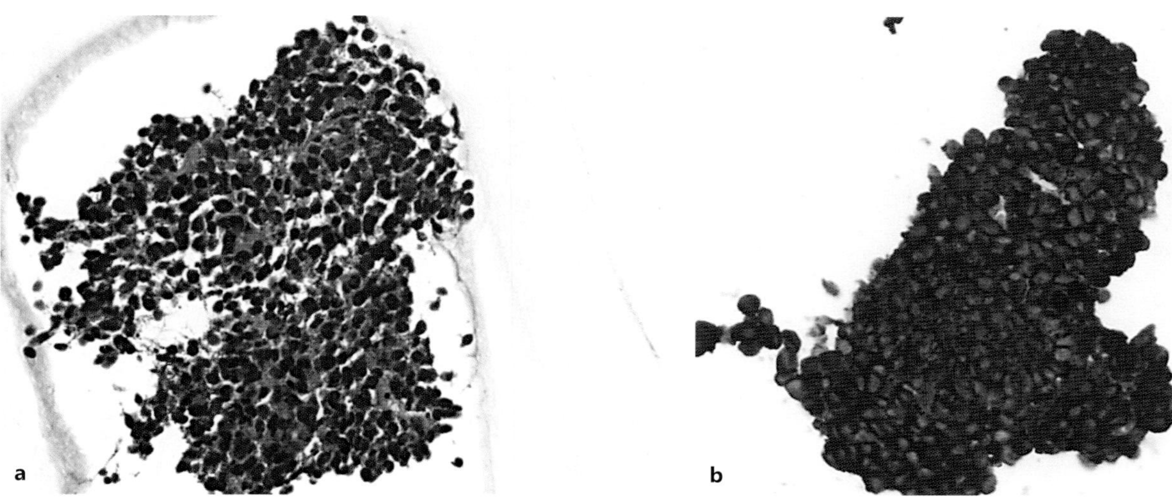

Fig. 6. Metastatic malignant melanoma. Amelanic melanomas cannot be reliably distinguished from breast cancer on the basis of morphology. A strong, diffuse positivity of the marker HMB-45 reveals the nature of this neoplasm. H&E (**a**) and cell block HMB-45 immunocytochemistry (**b**). Intermediate power.

tubular carcinomas with luminal A cancers, the choice of the right treatment is based on the expression of molecular prognostic and predictive markers. A recent study investigating the morphological features of triple-negative cancers on FNAC sample evidenced some distinctive traits of these neoplasms that were useful to differentiate between luminal A and B cancers, but they were unreliable for a distinction from HER2-overexpressing tumors [Akashi et al., 2013].

In our opinion molecular breast cancer subtypes are useful in the context of a multidisciplinary team, mainly to improve the communication with clinicians concerning the prognosis and the most appropriate management of breast cancer patients. Nevertheless, they must not replace the classical histotypes, which still represent independent prognostic factors and in some cases describe the behavior and peculiarities of neoplasms better than the molecular classification does.

References

Akashi S, Kuwabara H, Kurisu Y, Takahashi Y, Yasuda E, Takeshita A, Ishizaki S, Tsuji M, Shibayama Y: Fine-needle aspiration cytology of triple-negative basal-like breast cancer. Diagn Cytopathol 2013; 41:283–287.

Allred DC: Issues and updates: evaluating estrogen receptor-α, progesterone receptor and HER2 in breast cancer. Mod Pathol 2010;23(suppl 2):S52–S59.

Bauer KR, Brown M, Cress RD, Parise CA, Caggiano V: Descriptive analysis of estrogen receptor (ER)-negative, progesterone receptor (PR)-negative, and HER2-negative invasive breast cancer, the so-called triple-negative phenotype: a population-based study from the California Cancer Registry. Cancer 2007;109:1721–1728.

Beraki E, Sauer T: Determination of HER-2 status on FNAC material from breast carcinomas using in situ hybridization with dual chromogen visualization with silver enhancement (dual SISH). Cytojournal 2010;7:21.

Early Breast Cancer Trialists Collaborative Group (EBCTCG): Effects of chemotherapy and hormonal therapy for early breast cancer on recurrence and 15-year survival: an overview of the randomised trials. Lancet 2005;365:1687–1717.

Ferguson J, Chamberlain P, Cramer HM, Wu HH: ER, PR, and Her2 immunocytochemistry on cell-transferred cytologic smears of primary and metastatic breast carcinomas: a comparison study with formalin-fixed cell blocks and surgical biopsies. Diagn Cytopathol 2012;41:575–581.

Geyer FC, Pareja F, Weigelt B, Rakha E, Ellis IO, Schnitt SJ, Reis-Filho JS: The spectrum of triple-negative breast disease: high- and low-grade lesions. Am J Pathol 2017;187:2139–2151.

Hammond ME, Hayes DF, Dowsett M, Allred DC, Hagerty KL, Badve S, Fitzgibbons PL, Francis G, Goldstein NS, Hayes M, Micks DG, Lester S, Love R, Mangu PB, McShane L, Miller K, Osborne CK, Paik S, Perlmutter J, Rhodes A, et al: American Society of Clinical Oncology/College of American Pathologists guideline recommendations for immunohistochemical testing of estrogen and progesterone receptors in breast cancer. J Clin Oncol 2010;28:2784–2795.

Hanley KZ, Siddiqui MT, Lawson D, Cohen C, Nassar A: Evaluation of new monoclonal antibodies in detection of estrogen receptor, progesterone receptor, and Her2 protein expression in breast carcinoma cell block sections using conventional microscopy and quantitative image analysis. Diagn Cytopathol 2009;37:251–257.

Hennigs A, Riedel F, Marmé F, Sinn P, Lindel K, Gondos A, Smetanay K, Golatta M, Sohn C, Schuetz F, Heil J, Schneeweiss A: Changes in chemotherapy usage and outcome of early breast cancer patients in the last decade. Breast Cancer Res Treat 2016; 160:491–499.

Kinsella MD, Birdsong G, Siddiqui MT, Cohen C, Hanley KZ: Immunohistochemical detection of estrogen receptor, progesterone receptor and human epidermal growth factor receptor 2 in formalin-fixed breast carcinoma cell block preparations: correlation of results to corresponding tissue block (needle core and excision) samples. Diagn Cytopathol 2013;41:192–198.

Kocjan G, Bourgain C, Fassina A, Hagmar B, Herbert A, Kapila K, Kardum-Skelin I, Kloboves-Prevodnik V, Krishnamurthy S, Koutselini H, Majak B, Olszewski W, Onal B, Pohar-Marinsek Z, Shabalova I, Smith J, Tani E, Vielh P, Weiner H, Schenck U, et al: The role of breast FNAC in diagnosis and clinical management: a survey of current practice. Cytopathology 2008;19:271–278.

Lakhani SR, Ellis IO, Schnitt SJ, Tan PH, van de Vijver MJ (eds): World Health Organization classification of tumours of the breast; in World Health Organization Classification of Tumours. Lyon, IARC, 2012, vol 4.

Mygdakos N, Nikolaidou S, Tzilivaki A, Tamiolakis D: Liquid based preparation (LBP) cytology versus conventional cytology (CS) in FNA samples from breast, thyroid, salivary glands and soft tissues. Our experience in Crete (Greece). Rom J Morphol Embryol 2009;50:245–250.

Perou CM, Sorlie T, Eisen MB, Van de Rijn M, Jeffrey SS, Rees CA, Pollack JR, Ross DT, Johnsen H, Akslen LA, Fluge O, Pergamenschikov A, Williams C, Zhu SX, Lonning PE, Borresen-Dale AL, Brown PO, Botstein D: Molecular portraits of human breast tumours. Nature 2000;406:747–752.

Rodriguez C, Suciu V, Poterie A, Lacroix L, Miran I, Boichard A, Delaloge S, Deneuve J, Azoulay S, Mathieu MC, Valent A, Michiels S, Arnedos M, Vielh P: Concordance between HER-2 status determined by qPCR in Fine Needle Aspiration Cytology (FNAC) samples compared with IHC and FISH in Core Needle Biopsy (CNB) or surgical specimens in breast cancer patients. Mol Oncol 2016;10:1430–1436.

Rossi ED, Larghi A, Verna EC, et al: Endoscopic ultrasound-guided fine-needle aspiration with liquid-based cytologic preparation in the diagnosis of primary pancreatic lymphoma. Pancreas 2010;39: 1299–1302.

Shidham VB, Falzon M: Serous effusions; in Gray W, Kocjan G (eds): Diagnostic Cytopathology, ed 3. London, Elsevier, 2010, pp 139–143.

Symmans WF, Ayers M, Clark EA, Stec J, Hess KR, Sneige N, Buchholz TA, Krishnamurthy S, Ibrahim NK, Buzdar AU, Theriault RL, Rosales MF, Thomas ES, Gwyn KM, Green MC, Syed AR, Hortobagyi GN, Pusztai L: Total RNA yield and microarray gene expression profiles from fine-needle aspiration biopsy and core-needle biopsy samples of breast carcinoma. Cancer 2003;97:2960–2971.

Wolff AC, Hammond ME, Schwarty NJ, Hagerty KL, Allred DC, Cote RJ, Dowsett M, Fitzgibbons PL, Hanna WM, Langer A, McShane LM, Paik S, Pegram MD, Perez EA, Press MF, Rhodes A, Sturgeon C, Taube SE, Tubbs R, Vance GH, et al: American Society of Clinical Oncology/College of American Pathologists guideline recommendations for human epidermal growth factor receptor 2 testing in breast cancer. J Clin Oncol 2007;25: 118–145.

Pinamonti M, Zanconati F: Breast Cytopathology. Assessing the Value of FNAC in the Diagnosis of Breast Lesions.
Monogr Clin Cytol. Basel, Karger, 2018, vol 24, pp 113–114 (DOI: 10.1159/000479774)

Concluding Remarks

Fine-needle aspiration cytology (FNAC) has traditionally been regarded as the simplest, less invasive, and less expensive diagnostic procedure for the definition of breast lesions [Khemka et al. 2009; Saha et al. 2016; Wang et al., 2017]. In expert hands, it allows obtaining an accurate diagnosis in most breast lesions. The introduction of widespread mammographic screening programs and the consequent detection of a large number of small, nonpalpable lesions have increasingly established the routine use of other minimally invasive biopsy methods using heavier gauge cutting needles – core needle biopsies (CNBs) and other automatic, imaging-guided devices, such as vacuum-assisted biopsies – partially obscuring the central role of FNA [Brancato et al., 2012; Tabbara et al., 2000]. These new opportunities lead to a greater autonomy of the radiologists, who do not feel anymore the need of having the on-site cytopathologist attending the sampling session. Indeed, this professional is not always available in the "spoke" health care centers, although it is an indispensable element for the rapid on-site evaluation of sample adequacy and the "fast-track" diagnostic process. For this reason, CNB, previously considered as a second-level examination, available in cases with inadequate (C1) or indeterminate (C3–C4) cytology, has increasingly been used as a primary diagnostic method without resorting to cytology. Another reason for the spread of CNB in breast diagnostics is the possibility of performing the biomolecular analyses for the preoperative characterization of large tumors, which can benefit in some cases from neoadjuvant treatments. Recently, new recommendations propose to definitively abandon FNAC, restricting all morphological investigations to CNB [Willems et al., 2012].

But is this true? Has FNAC completely lost its role, allowing us to remove it from the routine diagnostic practice? After carefully reading the contemporary literature, it is evident that to this day FNAC maintains a role as first-level examination in all the centers where cytopathologists grant their constant presence in the radiology units: they take actively part in the sampling sessions, provide a clear and standardized report, including diagnostic categories, and integrate their diagnoses in the context of a multidisciplinary team [Berner et al., 2003; Brancato et al., 2012; Delaloge et al., 2016; Kocijan et al., 2008; Mitra and Dey, 2016]. This allows eventually completing the morphological diagnosis with ancillary techniques, when truly necessary, by resorting to further sampling. Moreover, this close collaboration between radiologist and pathologist leads to a better evaluation of the individual situation, and they decide together whether to extend the examination on multiple lesions and axillary lymph nodes, and eventually resort directly to CNB, if needed.

According to the current recommendations of the UK National Coordinating Committee for Breast Pathology [Lee et al., 2016], the use of FNAC should be limited principally to mass-forming breast lesions, whether clinically or radiologically evident, or for the evaluation of axillary lymph adenopathy. It is clear that FNAC should be proposed in centers where compliance to the quality standards is assured and can be demonstrated, as it is stated in the European guidelines [Perry et al., 2006]. Compliance to these standards allows accreditation of this method as first-choice diagnostic technique in certified breast unit centers, as also demonstrated by the experience of the Trieste Breast Unit. This is possible if an expert cytopathologist is available in the center, and if an adequate workload is assured, which should preferably be higher than 100–150 cases per year. Most important is the possibility of integrating the sample with supplementary material, especially when there is the possibility of a neoadjuvant treatment. Routine cytohistological comparison is critical to the maintenance of and for the improvement in diagnostic performance due its key role in the synthesis of preoperative diagnostic methods. A rational management of the diagnostic process of each patient and each lesion is possible only in the breast units where all diagnostic techniques, including FNAC, are available and meet the required quality criteria. In our personal experience from the Breast Unit of Trieste, where a systematic use of FNAC is available, it is proven that this method may result in a definitive diagnosis in 2/3 of the investigated lesions.

The unjustified abandonment of the technique by breast health care centers must be avoided, since it could only have negative repercussions on the whole preoperative diagnostic process. A reduced familiarity of pathologists with breast cytological samples could only negatively affect the ability to recognize also axillary lesions, for which FNAC is still widely used [Gipponi et al., 2016].

The advent of new molecular methods and the introduction of genomic sequencing should conversely increase the use of FNAC due to the undoubted quality advantage of cytological material compared with paraffin-embedded material. Thus, it is necessary for the pathologists to guarantee the maintenance of their professional expertise in this field and to transmit it to the young.

References

Berner A, Davidson B, Sigstad E, Risberg B: Fine-needle aspiration cytology vs core biopsy in the diagnosis of breast lesions. Diagn Cytopathol 2003;29:344–348.

Brancato B, Crocetti E, Bianchi S, Catarzi S, Risso GG, Bulgaresi P, Piscioli F, Scialpi M, Ciatto S, Houssami N: Accuracy of needle biopsy of breast lesions visible on ultrasound: audit of fine needle versus core needle biopsy in 3,233 consecutive samplings with ascertained outcomes. Breast 2012;21:449–454.

Delaloge S, Bonastre J, Borget I, Garbay JR, Fontenay R, Boinon D, Saghatchian M, Mathieu MC, Mazouni C, Rivera S, Uzan C, André F, Dromain C, Boyer B, Pistilli B, Azoulay S, Rimareix F, Bayou el-H, Sarfati B, Caron H, Ghouadni A, Leymarie N, Canale S, Mons M, Arfi-Rouche J, Arnedos M, Suciu V, Vielh P, Balleyguier C: The challenge of rapid diagnosis in oncology: diagnostic accuracy and cost analysis of a large-scale one-stop breast clinic. Eur J Cancer 2016;66:131–137.

Gipponi M, Fregatti P, Garlaschi A, Murelli F, Margarino C, Depaoli F, Baccini P, Gallo M, Friedman D: Axillary ultrasound and fine-needle aspiration cytology in the preoperative staging of axillary node metastasis in breast cancer patients. Breast 2016;30:146–150.

Khemka A, Chakrabarti N, Shah S, Patel V: Palpable breast lumps: fine-needle aspiration cytology versus histopathology: a correlation of diagnostic accuracy. Internet J Surg 2009;18:1.

Kocjan G, Bourgain C, Fassina A, Hagmar B, Herbert A, et al: The role of breast FNAC in diagnosis and clinical management: a survey of current practice. Cytopathology 2008;19:271–278.

Lee AHS, Anderson N, Carder P, Cooke J, Deb R, Ellis IO, Howe M, Jenkins JA, Knox F, Stephenson T, Shrimankar J, Wilson R: Non-Operative Diagnosis Working Group of the UK National Coordinating Committee for Breast Pathology. Guidelines for Non-Operative Diagnostic Procedures and Reporting in Breast Cancer Screening, June 2016. London, Royal College of Pathologists, 2017.

Mitra S, Dey P: Fine-needle aspiration and core biopsy in the diagnosis of breast lesions: a comparison and review of the literature. Cytojournal 2016;13:18.

Perry N, Broeders M, de Wolf C, Törnberg S, Holland R, von Karsa L, Puthaar E (eds): European Guidelines for Quality Assurance in Breast Cancer Screening and Diagnosis, ed 4. Luxembourg, European Commission, Office for Official Publications of the European Communities, 2006.

Saha A, Mukhopadhay M, Das C, Sarkar K, Saha AK, Sarkar DK: FNAC versus core needle biopsy: a comparative study in evaluation of palpable breast lump. J Clin Diagn Res 2016;10:EC05–EC08.

Tabbara SO, Frost AR, Stoler MH, Sneige N, Sidawy MK: Changing trends in breast fine-needle aspiration: results of the Papanicolaou Society of Cytopathology Survey. Diagn Cytopathol 2000;22:126–130.

Wang M, He X, Chang Y, Sun G, Thabane L: A sensitivity and specificity comparison of fine needle aspiration cytology and core needle biopsy in evaluation of suspicious breast lesions: a systematic review and meta-analysis. Breast 2017;31:157–166.

Willems SM, van Deurzen CH, van Diest PJ: Diagnosis of breast lesions: fine-needle aspiration cytology or core needle biopsy? A review. J Clin Pathol 2012;65:287–292.

Subject Index